Neuroscience Research Progress Series

# RELATIONSHIP BETWEEN AUTOMATIC AND CONTROLLED PROCESSES OF ATTENTION AND LEADING TO COMPLEX THINKING

# NEUROSCIENCE RESEARCH PROGRESS SERIES

**Dendritic Spines: Biochemistry, Modeling and Properties**
*Louis R. Baylog*
2009. ISBN: 978-1-60741-460-5

**Current Advances in Sleep Biology**
*Marcos G. Frank (Editor)*
2009. ISBN: 978-1-60741-508-4

**Relationship Between Automatic and Controlled Processes
of Attention and Leading to Complex Thinking**
*Rosa Angela Fabio*
2009: ISBN: 978-1-60741-810-8

Neuroscience Research Progress Series

# RELATIONSHIP BETWEEN AUTOMATIC AND CONTROLLED PROCESSES OF ATTENTION AND LEADING TO COMPLEX THINKING

## ROSA ANGELA FABIO

Nova Science Publishers, Inc.
*New York*

For permission to use material from this book please contact us:
Telephone 631-231-7269; Fax 631-231-8175
Web Site: http://www.novapublishers.com

## NOTICE TO THE READER

The Publisher has taken reasonable care in the preparation of this book, but makes no expressed or implied warranty of any kind and assumes no responsibility for any errors or omissions. No liability is assumed for incidental or consequential damages in connection with or arising out of information contained in this book. The Publisher shall not be liable for any special, consequential, or exemplary damages resulting, in whole or in part, from the readers' use of, or reliance upon, this material. Any parts of this book based on government reports are so indicated and copyright is claimed for those parts to the extent applicable to compilations of such works.

Independent verification should be sought for any data, advice or recommendations contained in this book. In addition, no responsibility is assumed by the publisher for any injury and/or damage to persons or property arising from any methods, products, instructions, ideas or otherwise contained in this publication.

This publication is designed to provide accurate and authoritative information with regard to the subject matter covered herein. It is sold with the clear understanding that the Publisher is not engaged in rendering legal or any other professional services. If legal or any other expert assistance is required, the services of a competent person should be sought. FROM A DECLARATION OF PARTICIPANTS JOINTLY ADOPTED BY A COMMITTEE OF THE AMERICAN BAR ASSOCIATION AND A COMMITTEE OF PUBLISHERS.

LIBRARY OF CONGRESS CATALOGING-IN-PUBLICATION DATA

Fabio, Rosa Angela.
  Relationship between automatic and controlled processes of attention and leading to complex thinking / author, Rosa Angela Fabio.
    p. cm.
  Includes bibliographical references and index.
  ISBN 978-1-60741-810-8 (hardcover)
  1. Attention. 2. Cognition. I. Title.
  [DNLM: 1. Attention. 2. Mental Processes. 3. Psychological Theory. 4. Thinking. BF 321 F118r 2009]
  BF321.F33 2009
  153.7--dc22
                                                                           2009018943

*Published by Nova Science Publishers, Inc. ✦ New York*

# CONTENTS

# PREFACE

This book begins with a theoretical and up-to-date overview on automatic and controlled processes. Automatic processing is effortless, fast and fairly error-free. It can be accomplished simultaneously with other cognitive processes without interference, it is not limited by attention capacity and it can be unconscious or involuntary. Controlled processing is effortful, slow and prone to errors but – at the same time, flexible and useful to deal with new tasks. Some automatic processes are thought to be pre-programmed or innate and include the encoding of temporal or spatial relationships, frequent monitoring and the activation of word meaning. Other cognitive processes become automatic with practice.

The second part deals the shift from controlled to automatic processing as the core of the access to complex thinking. When somebody starts learning, attention is allocated in order to fulfil task requirements. Performance requires controlled processing. When training proceeds, performance requires less vigilance, it becomes faster and faster and errors decrease. This is defined *automatization.* Automatization concerns both perceptual and motor skills and cognitive processes. The essence of the book is that high load in the coding of the stimuli results in reduced perception of distractor stimuli because there is insufficient capacity to process them all. The controlled processes can rely on and negatively influence higher mental functions, such as working memory, which are required to maintain current priorities and to choose between them, and also rely on complex thinking because this latter ask for an efficient working memory system.

Rosa Angela Fabio[*],
Department of Educational and Psychological Science,
University of Messina, Messina, Italy

---

[*] Correspondence to: Rosa Angela Fabio Ph.D, Professor of Psychology, Department of Educational and Psychological Science, University of Messina, Via Concezione 16, 98100 Messina, Tel. 39-339-3830770, e-mail: rafabio@unime.it

# INTRODUCTION

People have always understood that there are functions of their body that they are unable to control, even if they would like to. Examples may be the beating of the heart and breathing, activities that continue whether we want them to or not. Early mention of the term "automatic" was in reference to bodily functions, rather than to any psychological process such as perception, reasoning, or behavior. Only with the birth of psychology as a science - that is to say, only for the past 100 years of intellectual history - has the mind been considered and analyzed as an internal bodily organ, instead of a soul or spiritual essence.

Today it is well known that automaticity is an important phenomenon in everyday mental life. Many routine activities are performed quickly and effortlessly with little thought, in short, automatically. As a result, we often perform those activities on "automatic pilot" and turn our minds to other things. For example, we can order things on the table while conversing with our daughter or we can drive while considering the organization of our daily activities.

On the other hand, in everyday life we continually experience difficulties in performing complex tasks. These require the division, allocation and re-allocation of attention, depending on task demands and our currently active goals and intentions. In this case, the requested ability is not automatic but rather a controlled process.

As the main theories suggest, automatic processing is fast, effortless, autonomous, stereotypic, unavailable to conscious awareness and fairly error-free. It can be accomplished simultaneously with other cognitive processes without interference, it is not limited by attentional capacity and it can be unconscious or involuntary. Controlled processing is effortful, slow and prone to errors but – at the same time, flexible and useful to deal with novel situations.

The distinction between automatic and controlled processes is particularly important because both support behaviour that achieves goals and ultimately promotes survival. As Schneider and Chein (2003) underline, dual processing mechanisms would likely not have evolved unless there were survival advantages to having both modes of processing. They propose that automatic and controlled processing are two qualitatively different forms of processing that provide complementary benefits. The authors make a simulation of their assumption and they conclude that a single process alone cannot provide both the fast learning of controlled processing and the robust high speed parallel processing of automatic processing. So, although it may be less parsimonious to assume two different modes of processing, they argue that there are sufficient survival advantages to a two-process system over a unitary architecture to have allowed a dual process system to evolve.

The survival advantages to having both controlled and automatic processing are analogous to the non-overlapping and overlapping benefits of having rod and cone vision. With controlled processing:

- the fundamentals of new skills can be acquired quickly
- critical stimuli can be attended while ignoring normally relevant stimuli
- variables that allow general operations to be applied to temporarily relevant stimuli can take place
- learning can be passed between individuals by instruction or observation
- goal-directed behavior can be planned and executed

However, due to the slow execution, high effort, and poor robustness of controlled processing, it can operate on only a small number of stimuli at any time, and any skill acquired during controlled performance may not be sufficiently robust to resist rapid decay or deterioration in the presence of stressors. Despite taking a long time to acquire, automatic processing has the advantages of being robust under stress, leading to long-term retention of associated skills, and allowing many processes to occur at high speed.

The aim of the present book is to study in depth these processes and to show that they are the core of learning and adaption.

The book is divided into two parts. The first contains four chapters that address the present theoretical questions about these two processes. The second contains application fields, in which it is shown that controlled and automatic processing are not merely interesting topics for cognitive psychologists to research. They also have consequences for many of a person's phenomenal experiences.

We begin, in chapter one, with a theoretical and up-to-date overview concerning automatic and controlled processes. The definitions of automatic and controlled processes will be provided, then a brief history of the early development of scientific approaches to automatic and controlled processes will be presented, followed by more in-depth examinations of the major strands in contemporary twentieth and twenty first century research. Since the field of automatization deals with both mnestic and attentional factors, in this book mnemonic and attentional theoretical contribution will be discussed.

In chapter two the major empirical paradigms in which these phenomena are explored are will be presented. Initially the search paradigm is presented, afterward the Stroop task and the priming paradigm are presented. Afterward Merrill procedure with a visual search paradigm is analyzed and finally the clock test of Moron. In the concluding section some thoughts about the relationship between different paradigm are offered.

In chapter three the growing body of functional anatomical studies, which examine the brain structures activated in the context of controlled and automatic behaviour will be addressed. This line of enquiry represents an important development in clarifying the construct of automaticity.

An account of the neural pathways involved in automatic processing will also be proposed. This approach involving the examination of functional imaging studies and possible neural circuitry will speak to the issue of whether automatic processing is quantitatively different (in the form of faster neural activity) from controlled processing or whether it differs qualitatively (utilising different strategies).

The first part of the book ends with a question regarding the costs and benefits of controlled and automatic processes that is proposed in chapter four. The utility and limitations of automatization will be discussed.

Beginning in the second part of the book, chapter five will explore ways of accessing complex thinking through automatization. It is suggested that with training, people can operate attentional control and improve their logical abilities.

The theme of operational implications (utility in empowerment of logical ability) continues in Chapter six, when we consider that controlled and automatic processing are not merely topics of academic interest to cognitive psychologists. They have very serious consequences for a person's phenomenal experience (such as to the degree to which one has control over one's emotions) and for one's relations with others (such as whether one's opinions and treatment of them is biased). They relate to the way in which attitudes form and change, to the way in which inner states are expressed to others, and by implication, to one's degree of free will in obeying authority, conforming to others, and reacting to people in need of help.

The second part of the book ends with the clinical point of view and with the application of both concepts, automatic and controlled processes, on clinical populations. In effect in chapter seven these processes are analysed with reference to the ability of learning disabled children and to the way in which they can learn. The chapter ends with the analysis of excess of automatization in anxiety, depression and addictive behaviours.

# PART I:
# THE ROLE OF AUTOMATIC AND CONTROLLED PROCESSES ON COGNITION

*Chapter 1*

# A THEORETICAL OVERVIEW ON AUTOMATIC AND CONTROLLED COGNITIVE PROCESSES

## ABSTRACT

The purpose of this chapter is to present a theoretical and up to date overview on automatic and controlled processes. Initially the definitions of automatic and controlled processes are provided. The main characteristics of automatic and controlled processes and the four meanings of automatic process are emphasised. The four meaning refers to the way in which some actions are carried out, to the way in which some actions are initiated without any conscious deliberation, to the orienting response and to the cases where tasks can be combined without any apparent interference. Main theoretical issues on the automatic/controlled processes are discussed. They concern the relationship between automatic and preattentive processes, conscious control, continuum of automatic and controlled processes, computational similarity and the fastness of automatic processes in comparison with controlled processes. Afterwards a brief history of the early development of scientific approaches to automatic and controlled processes is presented, followed by more in-depth examinations of the contemporary major strands in twentieth century research. In the concluding section some thoughts are offered about the relationship between scientific progress and everyday understanding of both processes.

## ON DEFINING AUTOMATIC AND CONTROLLED PROCESSES

There has been followed an extended effort to develop an empirical and theoretical understanding of automatic and controlled processing [1, 2, 3, 4].

As the main theories suggest automatic processing is fast [5, 6], effortless [2, 7], autonomous [2, 6, 7, 8], stereotypic [9], unavailable to conscious awareness [10] and fairly error-free. It can be accomplished simultaneously with other cognitive processes without interference, it is not limited by attention capacity and it can be unconscious or involuntary. Controlled processing is effortful, slow and prone to errors but – at the same time, flexible and useful to deal with new tasks.

As Norman & Shallice [11] underline, automatic process has at least four meanings. First, it refers to the way in which some actions are carried out without awareness: for example, walking on an even surface. Second, it refers to the way in which some actions are initiated without any conscious deliberation, such as sipping a drink while talking. Third, attention may be automatically drawn to a stimulus, as in the orienting response to a sudden onset of a visual signal in the periphery [12]. Last, automatic control is used to refer to the cases where tasks can be combined without any apparent interference, difference or competition for processing resources.

Controlled processing is deliberate and conscious and can deal with only a limited amount of information at once. When tasks interfere, this is usually taken to indicate competition for limited attentional processing resources. Conscious control requires attention: automatic control does not.

There are some interesting theoretical issues on the automatic/controlled discussion. They concern relationship between automatic and preattentive processes, conscious control, continuum of automatic and controlled processes, computational similarity and the fastness of automatic processes in comparison with controlled processes.

The first issue concerns the relationship between automatic and preattentive processes. Despite the fact that automatic processes are described as very similar to preattentive processes in that both, by definition, occur in the absence of attention, Treisman et al. [13] note, however, that there are many important differences.

First, automatic and preattentive processes become independent from attention in different ways. While automatic processes are developed through extended practice, preattentive processes are governed by mechanisms that are either innate or acquired early in life. In addition, automatic and preattentive processes are functionally different. Automatic processes support skilled behaviour; in many experiments, after much practice, the subjects show dramatic improvement in performing two tasks at the same time [15]; preattentive processes support low-level perceptual functions such as feature detection.

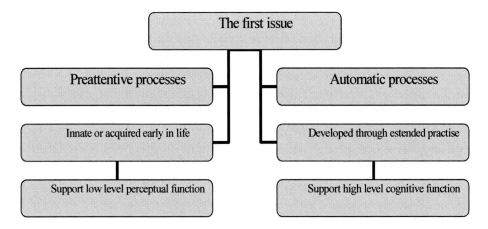

Figure 1. Table of the differences between preattentive and automatic processes

The second issue concerns conscious control. Control is often (explicitly or implicitly) equated to conscious control. Umiltà and Moscovitch [16], who are proponents of this view, suggest that consciousness embodies the function of control, and that voluntary control over cognitive processes depend on the phenomenal experience of being conscious. The fact that we have phenomenal experience of a process brings it under voluntary control.

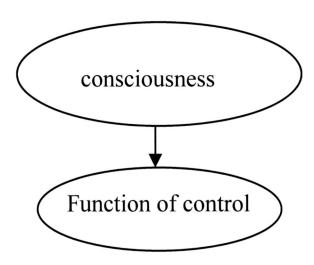

Figure 2. The Umiltà and Moscovitch's view

The third issue involves the continuum of automatic and controlled processes. The above presented dichotomy between "controlled" and "automatic" processing firstly appeared in the influential paper by Schneider and Shiffrin [7]. With reference to this dichotomy, in automatic mode, processing is a passive outcome of stimulation; it is parallel and does not draw on attentional capacity. In conscious control mode, mental processing is consciously controlled by intentions and draws on attentional capacity. Today, however, this dichotomy has been softened by use, so that "automaticity" may now be seen more as a matter of degree than as an all-or- none state.

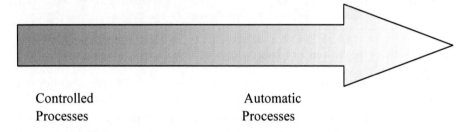

Controlled                           Automatic
Processes                            Processes

Figure 3. Continuum of controlled and automatic processes

Although as noted several theorists, defined automatic processes as being attention free, unconscious, and involuntary, it is rarely the case, however, for all three features to hold simultaneously [17, 18]. Bargh [19] pointed out that the ability of a process to run to completion once started, without the need of conscious monitoring, is common to all automatic processes, and Tzelgov [20] proposed the adoption of processing without monitoring as the definition of automaticity. A process is automatic if it has (due to genetic prewiring or due to routinization by practice; [2, 21, 21]) acquired the ability to run without monitoring. Once a process has been automatized it can be performed automatically as part of the task requirements, by being a component of a higher order processing scheme defined by the required task (see Vallacher & Wegner [23]. Or, it can run in an autonomous mode, as happens in Stroop-like phenomena and in the Exclusion task in the process dissociation paradigm [24]. Tzelgov [20] pointed out that the defining condition for the automaticity of a process is that it can run in the autonomous mode.

The fourth issue is the assumption that automatic processes are computationally similar but faster than controlled processes.

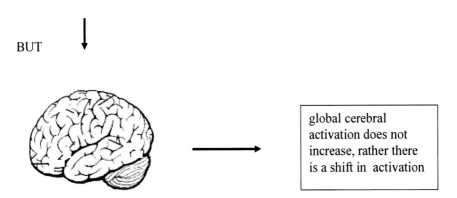

Figure 4. The Saling and Phillips's view

As Saling and Phillips [25] point out, automatic processes, rather than merely being faster than controlled processes, are instead economical and elegant, occurring without uncertainty or hesitation. Although automaticity is seemingly faster at a behavioural level, in the form of more efficient behaviour, this cannot be equated with faster processing at a neural level. Their paper outlines functional anatomical evidence supporting the position that automatic processes are qualitatively different from controlled processes. As the authors underline if automaticity indeed involved faster processing, one would expect to see more processing as reflected by increased global cerebral activation with the acquisition of automaticity. Instead, there is a decrease in global activation or a shift in activation, particularly from cortical regions to subcortical areas. Thus, automatic processing is performed differently from controlled processing, apparently employing different, superior algorithms, which in some cases are explicit and in other cases are yet to be documented.

In the specific literature, there can be other words used to refer to automatic and controlled processes that are discussed below:

- Reflexes and voluntary behaviour
- Exogenous and endogenous attention control
- top-down and bottom-up processes
- stimulus driven and voluntary driven
- declarative and procedural memory
- serial and parallel processing

Reflexes, at one extreme, occur in direct response to certain classes of stimuli unless actively inhibited (a light in the eye causes the restriction of the pupil). At the other extreme are voluntary behaviors such as deciding what to do in a difficult moment [26]

Posner's [27] distinction between exogenous and endogenous attention controls, stated that exogenous control is explicitly modeled on the neurological concept of a reflex and that attention control lies outside the organism, namely in the stimuli impinging on the organism. If the appropriate stimulus arises, the response of attending to that stimulus will occur. In endogenous control, control lies inside the organism. Thus, whereas exogenous attention control is characterized as stimulus driven, endogenous control is typically characterized as cognitively driven.

Because of the key role attributed to the stimulus, exogenous control has often been characterized as stimulus-driven or bottom-up control. In the other hypothesized mode of attention control (endogenous/nonautomatic/voluntary), control is thought to reflect the same sort of decisions that we make to initiate any other (overt) voluntary action. Whereas a cognitive decision is hypothesized to be necessary for an endogenous attention shift, no particular stimulus event is necessary for the exogenous.

Declarative memory (working memory) is severely limited in the amount of information that can be concurrently represented in it. Procedural memory is not limited.

"Serial" refers to the way of processing implied by the conscious activity. Since consciousness has a limited capacity system, it is serial. On the other hand, parallel refers to the way of processing implied by the automatic activity, free of limits, and so, executable in parallel mode.

In this book the preferred reference is to automatic and controlled processing.

In the following part of this chapter historical and up to date theories of automatic and controlled processes will be introduced. With reference to historical contributions, Atkinson and Shiffrin model [28], Posner and Snyder [6] and Shiffrin and Schneider's [7] theories will be presented. With reference to up to date contributions, Neuman's critique of the two-process theory, Gopher's suggestions about control, Anderson's theory, Logan's model, Norman and Shallice's model, and Pasler's theory will be presented.

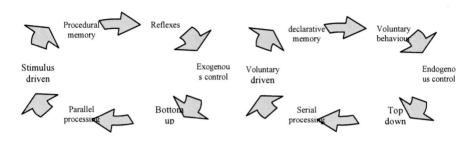

Figure 5. The two ways of automatic and controlled processes

## Theories of Automatic and Controlled Processing

With reference to historical contributions, a recent book of Styles [29] enlightens the view of different authors; she starts with a memory model. Atkinson and Shiffrin [28] pointed out the importance of understanding not only the structure of the information processing system, but also how it was controlled. In Atkinson and Shiffrin's model the selection, rehearsal and recoding of information in short-term memory all required control processes. Short-term memory was seen as a working memory in which both storage and processing took place. The more demanding the processing was, the less capacity would be available for storage and vice versa. Atkinson and Shiffrin tell us nothing about this control, except that it is something that the subject does.

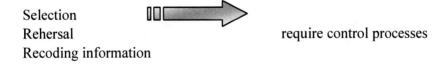

Selection
Rehersal                                                        require control processes
Recoding information

Figure 6. The Atkinson and Shiffrin's view

Posner and Snyder [6] drew the distinction between automatic activation processes which are solely the result of past learning and processes that are under current conscious control: Automatic activation processes are those which may occur without intention, without any conscious awareness and without interference with other mental activity. They are distinguished from operations that are performed by the conscious processing system since the latter of limited capacity and thus its commitments to any operation reduce its availability to perform any other operation. Posner and Snyder were interested in the extent to which our conscious intentions and strategies are in control of the way information is processed in our minds. They thought that the conscious processing system was a general purpose limited capacity system because they sad that any attention demand of one task would reduce the amount of attention available for another attention demanding task.

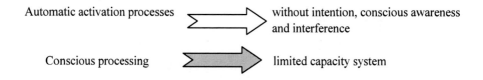

Automatic activation processes ⟹ without intention, conscious awareness and interference

Conscious processing ⟹ limited capacity system

Figure 7. The Posner and Snyder's view

Another general theory involving controlled and automatic processing was proposed by Schneider and Shiffrin [7] who caried out a series of experiments on visual search and attention. In one experiment performance was tested when subjects had to search for a member of the memory set in visual displays containing one, two, or four items. Their task was to decide as rapidly as possible whether any of the letters from the memory set were present in the display. The crucial experimental manipulation was the mapping between stimuli and responses. For the *consistent mapping* condition, targets were always consonants and distractors were always digits i.e., there was a consistent mapping of target and distractors onto their responses. In this case, whenever the subject detected a member of the memory set in the display, it had to be a target. Performance in the consistent mapping condition was contrasted with that called *varied mapping* condition. In this condition both the memory set and the distractors were a mixture of letters and digits. Schneider and Shiffrin found a clear difference between performances in the two conditions. With consistent mapping, search is virtually independent of both the number of items in the memory set and the number of items in the display, as if search is taking place in parallel. Schneider and Shiffrin [7] said this type of performance reflected "automatic processing". However, with varied mapping where the target and distractor set changed from trial to trial, subjects were slower to detect the target and their response times increased with the number of distractors in the display. Search seemed to remain serial. This type of performance was said to be indicative of "controlled processing".

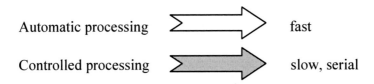

Figure 8. The Shiffrin and Schneider's view

An author that criticizes all the two-process theories is Neuman [17]. He summarises the criteria of automaticity on which most two process theories agree, under three headings:

1. Mode of operation: Automatic processes operate without capacity and they neither suffer nor cause interference.
2. Mode of control: Automatic processes are under the control of stimulation rather than under the control of the intentions (strategies, expectancies, plans) of the person.
3. Mode of representation: Automatic processes do not necessarily give rise to conscious awareness.

Some "secondary criteria"—which do not necessarily define automaticity but which are suggested or implied by some theories—are that automatic processes are determined by connections that are either wired in or are learned through practice: and that this kind of processing is relatively simple, rapid, and inflexible in that it can be modified only by extended practice.

Neuman then goes on to evaluate the data to try to determine whether these criteria are correct, and then to specify the functional properties of automatic and non-automatic processes. He argues that an automatic processing task can require attentional capacity. While a controlled processing task may be "interference free" in one task combination, in a different combination, interference may well be found—hence, the task now appears to require attention while before it did not. Literature shows that processing of the unwanted stimulus dimension will be "automatic" only within a constrained set of circumstances, when the subject's ability to focus attention breaks down. Neuman suggests that distractors produce interference not simply because they are present in the stimulus environment, but because they are related to the intended action. Neuman admits that there probably are situations in which stimulus processing may be unavoidable, and outside the control of current intentions, and believes that automatic processing is not uncontrolled, but rather is controlled below the level of conscious awareness. Awareness is one of the key properties of conscious control. But what do we mean by awareness, or consciousness, for that matter?

In Neuman's analysis there are three kinds of unawareness. He says there are three questions we can ask and particularly whether brain processes not directly related to ongoing activity are "unaware" whether there are some processes within the execution of a task that may escape awareness and whether an action as a whole can proceed without awareness. Neuman replies affirmatively to all the three questions, and proposes a different conception of automaticity: he suggests that the difference between automatic and controlled processing is the level of control required.

Automatic processing

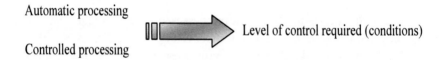 Level of control required (conditions)

Controlled processing

Figure 9. The Neuman's view

Actions can be performed only if all the parameters for that action are specified. Some parameter specifications are stored in long-term memory; Neuman terms these parameters "skills". Other specifications come from the stimulus itself, but the remaining specifications must come from an attentional mechanism, whose function is to provide the specifications that cannot be obtained by linking input information to skills.

According to Neuman, skills have two functions. First, they specify actions and secondly they help pick up information from the environment. Thus, according to Neuman (1984) a process is automatic if its parameters are specified by a skill in conjunction with input information. If this is not possible, one or several attentional mechanisms for parameter specification must come into play. They are responsible for interference and give rise to conscious awareness. It is clear from Neuman's argument that automaticity is not some kind of process, but something that seems to emerge when conditions are right. The right conditions depend not only on the processing system but also on the situation.

Gopher focuses on the strategies that allow us to cope with competing task demands within the boundaries of our processing and response limitations. Given that we are able to adopt and execute attentional strategies, Gopher asks three further questions about control: the first is to what extent we can be consciously aware of the strategies we use and their efficiency; the second how we do it; and the third how changes in attentional strategy are implemented.

As an example in focused attention experiments, subjects do focus attention as far as they are able within the context of the experiment. In divided attention experiments subjects are able to divide attention, and can do so according to priorities. If one ask subjects to give 70% attention to one task and 30% to another task, they can usually become able to do this.

After a series of experiments on training on attentional control, Gopher enlightens that the skill of attentional control appears to be learned. Gopher suggests that there is a move from controlled application of attentional strategies to automated schemata, where response schemata that have become associated with proficient behaviour become hard-wired. With learning, the attentional strategies that once needed control become automatic.

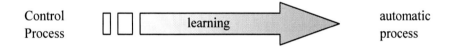

Control Process | learning | automatic process

Figure 10. The Gopher's view

Anderson's (1983) and Logan's (1998) theories relate automaticity to mnemonic aspects of attention rather than to resource limitations.

Anderson (1983) provides a theory of cognition based on a production system called "Encoding Processes and the Action of Productions". An important distinction made by memory theorists is between declarative knowledge, to which we have conscious access, and procedural knowledge, to which we have no conscious access. This distinction between procedural and declarative knowledge is fundamental in the model of Anderson. Working memory (declarative) is severely limited in the amount of information that can be concurrently represented in it. If all the computational steps involved in human information processing had to be represented in declarative form in working memory, the system would be in danger of overload. However, if only a small amount of task-relevant information needed to be represented in declarative form, the system could run much more efficiently. Provided the declarative system has access to the outputs from productions, there is no need for the productions themselves to be open to conscious inspection.

Like Freud at the beginning of the XXth century, Allport [48, 49] and Neuman [17] suggest that only a very small amount of information processing is available to consciousness, and that unconscious processing is the rule rather than the exception. Productions in Anderson's ACT model run off automatically as products of their execution enter working memory.

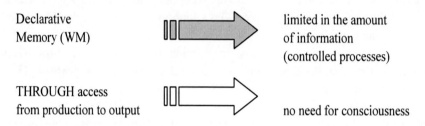

| Declarative Memory (WM) | | limited in the amount of information (controlled processes) |

| THROUGH access from production to output | | no need for consciousness |

Figure 11. The Anderson's view

Also Logan's theory relates automaticity to memorial aspeccts of attention rather than to resource limitations. Automaticity is seen as memory retrieval: performance is automatic when based on single-step direct access retrieval of past solutions from memory. Novices begin with a general algorithm that is sufficient to perform the task. As they gain experience, they respond with the solution retrieved from memory. The theory makes three main assumptions:

1. coding into memory is an obligatory consequence of attention
2. the retrieval from memory is an obligatory, unavoidable consequence of attention
3. each encounter with a stimulus is encoded, stored and retrieved separately

This theory is called "instance theory". These assumptions imply a learning mechanism that produces a gradual transition from algorithmic processing to memory-based processing. The assumption of obligatory retrieval is supported by studies of Stroop and primimg effects, in which attention to an item activates associations in memory that facilitate performance in some situations and interfere with it in others [30] . The instance theory implies also that the automatization is item-based rather than process-based. It implies that automatization involves learning specific responses to specific stimuli.

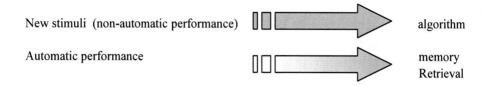

New stimuli (non-automatic performance)  algorithm

Automatic performance  memory Retrieval

Figure 12. The Logan's view

Due to this specificity, transfer to novel stimuli and situations should be poor. By contrast the modal view suggests that automatization is process-based, making the underlyng processes more efficient, reducing the amount of resources required or the number of steps to be executed.   The theory differs from process based views of automatization in that it assumes that a task is performed differently when is automatic and when it is not. Automatic performance is based on memory retrieval, whereas non-automatic performance is based on an algorithm.

Recently Boronat & Logan [31] try to specify at what level attention operates in automatization. In their research, authors investigated whether attention operates in the encoding of automatized information, the retrieval of automatized information, or in both cases. Subjects searched two-word displays for members of a target category in focused-attention or divided-attention conditions that were crossed with block (training vs. transfer). To see whether subjects encoded all available items or only attended items, they compared performance for subjects in different training conditions but in the same transfer condition. Subjects encoded attended items. To see whether subjects retrieved all the items they had in memory, or only items associated with that to which they were attending at retrieval, they compared performance for subjects in the same training conditions but in different transfer conditions. Subjects retrieved attended items. Attention was found to operate at both encoding and retrieval. These findings support the instance theory of automaticity, which predicts the role of attention at encoding and retrieval.

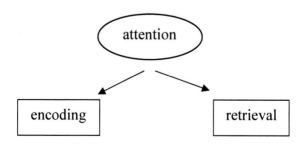

Figure 13. The Boronat and Logan's view

Also Treisman proposes a theory that is related with the Logan Model. Treisman deals with automaticity with reference to preattentive processing.

Treisman and Treisman et al. [32, 33] suggest that preattentive processing is a bottom-up process which reflects the activation of populations of feature detectors. To the extent that automatic and preattentive processes are governed by the same underlying mechanisms, automaticity might reflect the build up of such detectors. If true, the transfer of automaticity to other tasks that reflect preattentive processing would be expected. Treisman et al. investigated this possibility by training subjects in two visual search tasks, and then, after sufficient practice, by seeing whether the targets were detected as rapidly in tasks thought to require preattentive processing. The transfer tasks were a motion detection task and figure ground separation task. Briefly, Treisman et al. found little evidence for transfer. Furthermore, minor changes in the visual search task (e.g., changing the color of the background) disrupted performance. Treisman et al. explain these findings in terms of Logan's instance theory.

According to feature theory, attention is not required for the detection of simple features, although attention shifts to these features once detected. To illustrate, deciding whether there is a red O among green Os does not require that attention be focused on the red O. Detection is preattentive. By contrast, attention is required for the conjunction of features. For example, attention must be focused on the target stimulus if the task is to locate a blue Q among red Qs and blue and red Os. Memory traces for conjunctive targets should therefore contain more specific information, such as spatial location. Treisman et al. tested this by contrasting visual search for feature and conjunctive targets. In both experiments, two of the four feature targets appeared in two spatial locations on 75% of the trials; the other two targets were equally likely to appear in any of the eight spatial locations.

Treisman, Vieira & Hayes [33] calculated costs and benefits of consistent targets appearing in consistent and inconsistent locations were defined relative to inconsistent targets appearing in random locations. The costs and benefits were greater for conjnctive targets (a blue Q among red Qs and blue and red Os) than for feature targets (e.g., a blue Q among red Qs). Furthermore, in conjunctive search but not in feature search, there was a small benefit for inconsistent targets appearing in consistent locations when they were the same color as the consistent target, or shared one dimension in common. This suggests that the build-up of position specific traces accounts well for speed up in conjunctive search, but not in feature search. The trace seems to be a conjunction of color, form, and location.

To summarize up to this point, while preattentive and automatic processes are similar in that both occur in the absence of attention, the origin of independence from attention for these processes seems to differ. Consistently with Logan's instance theory, automaticity, but not preattentive processing, seems to be mediated by the buildup of position-specific memory traces. Treisman et al. [33] suggest that the origin of independence for preattentive processes is populations of feature detectors.

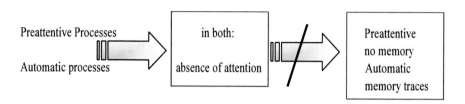

Figure 14. The Treisman's view

The results of Treisman et al. suggest that automaticity in conjunctive search is mediated by the build up of memory traces that consist of conjunctions of location, color, and dimension. Unitization of conjunctions into preattentively available features would results in zero slopes. An alternative possibility, therefore, is that the comparison process becomes more rapid and efficient. By other criteria, search became automatic. For example, scanning for targets shifted from voluntary to involuntary.

The models above presented refer mainly to automatization. On the other extreme some other authors try to understand controlled behaviours. In this line, Styles [29] refers to Norman and Shallice's model of willed and automatic control of behaviour.

Norman and Shallice (1986) propose that there are a number of different kinds of tasks that require deliberate attentional resources and propose that these are needed when tasks:

1. Require planning or decision making.
2. Involve components of trouble shooting.
3. Are ill-learned or contain novel sequences.
4. Are judged to be dangerous or technically difficult.
5. Require overcoming a strong habitual response.

Norman and Shallice attempt to account for a variety of phenomena concerning controlled and automatic behaviour. For example, some action sequences that normally run off automatically can be earned out under conscious control if needed, so deliberate conscious control can suppress unwanted actions and facilitate wanted actions. In the Stroop color the unwanted action "Name the word" (automatic) can be suppressed (by deliberate conscious control) in order to "Name the colour". This example is one that falls into the "overcoming habitual response" category.

Their theoretical framework centres around the idea that we have action schemata in long-term memory which are awaiting the appropriate set of conditions to be triggered.

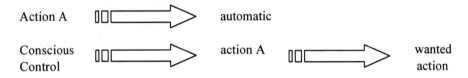

Figure 15. The Norman and Shallice's view

Normally, the most strongly activated schema will take control of action. In the Stroop example, this would be the written word. However, for the colour to be named, there must be attentional biasing of the schema for or naming the colour that allows the normally weaker response to become the most active schema and gain control of action.

There are then, two sources of activation, one from the stimulus environment which acts bottom-up and another which acts top-down according to the current goal. An important component of the model is a basic mechanism called "contention scheduling". This sorts out conflicting schemata by interactive inhibition and excitation. The operation of this system is similar to the interactive activation model of letter recognition proposed by McClelland and Rumelhart [34].

Recently the SAS has been equated with the central executive in Baddeley's [35] model of working memory. Unlike Broadbent [38], who tried to avoid the homunculus problem in his Maltese Cross model of memory by proposing control resulted from the operation of productions, Baddeley posits control by the SAS [36, 37]. This is, however, a homunculus by a different name. By giving control over to the SAS, Norman and Shallice [11] and Baddeley [35] seem to have done little more than re-name "the subject" in Atkinson and Skiffrin's [28] model of short-term memory as "the supervisory attentional system". However, Baddeley [35] believes that the homunculus can serve a useful purpose provided that we remember it is a way of labelling a problem rather than explaining it and that we continue to work at "stripping away the various functions we previously attributed to our homunculus until eventually it can be declared redundant". Baddeley points out that whether the central executive will prove to be a single unitary system or a number of autonomous control processes is yet to be discovered. Certainly there is good evidence that people act as if they have an SAS and can behave in goal-directed ways, initiating and changing behaviours, apparently at will.

The symptoms of frontal lobe patients are well explained in terms of Norman and Shallice's [11] model. Indeed, it is patient data that has provided a large part of the data on which these authors based their ideas. If the SAS is damaged, it will be unable to bias the schemata which are intended to control action, or switch from a currently active schema (current mental-set) to a new one. The inability to change the schema which is currently controlling action would produce perseveration errors, as in the Wisconsin cardsorting test. Further, if the SAS is out of action, the schema most strongly activated by the environmental cues, will capture control of action, as in the example of R.J. cutting string, and would explain impulsive, "uncontrolled" behaviour. An interesting point to note here is, that although the patient can tell you what they should be doing (i.e. *not* cutting string) the verbal information has no impact on behaviour. So although at a conscious level the patient "knows" what to do, at another, unconscious level, the information processing does not know.

In the previous part of the chapter we saw separately automatic and controlled processes. Pashler [26] complicates both fields. He shows that the phenomenon of involuntary attention capture, often presumed to be entirely bottom-up and stimulus driven, turns out to be subtly influenced by top-down goals. He shows also that attention capture, a phenomenon that appears at first glance to be entirely under top-down cognitive control, turns out to be heavily influenced by bottom-up, stimulus-driven processing.

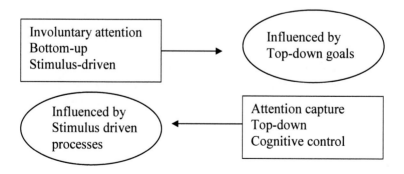

Figure 16. The Pashler's view

Pashler stated also that one of the key properties attributed to the exogenous or reflexive mode of attention control is that it is involuntary. That is, attention capture depends only on the occurrence of the proper stimulus, not on the goals of the observer. Visual search times decrease with abrupt-onset targets and increase with abrupt-onset distractors even when, across trials, the location of abrupt onset stimuli is unrelated with the location of the target (e.g. Yantis & Jonides 1990, Mueller & Rabbitt 1989). Thus, it was argued that abrupt-onset stimuli can capture attention independently of the will of the subject.

By the early 1990s there appeared to be a broad consensus that the reflexive mode of attention control is free of influence from top-down cognitive processes. According to this view, attentional control is at the mercy of the appearance of certain classes of stimuli (be they transients, abrupt-onset stimuli, new objects, or more generally, relatively salient stimuli). Such stimuli would draw attention in a completely bottom-up manner, overriding or at least delaying the cognitively driven, top-down control of attention.

Yantis & Jonides [39] however, noted one special case in which voluntary processes could prevent capture. If subjects know with certainty the location of a target and are given sufficient time to focus attention on that target, then distractor stimuli are at least momentarily unable to capture attention (see also Theeuwes, [40]). This finding suggests that if an observer's attention is already locked onto one location, the power of other stimuli to draw attention is nullified. (It is unclear whether this nullification occurs because perceptual processing of the distractors is prevented, or due to a "lock-up" of the attention-shifting mechanism, which prevents a new shift.) In any event, this exception appears restricted to situations in which attention is tightly focussed on a object.

Pashler conclude that it is certainly the case that serial and parallel models may mimic each other in certain contexts, particularly with respect to patterns of mean response times [41]. However, a variety of techniques now exist for successfully distinguishing these types of processes, and the question of whether different sorts of mental events can or cannot operate simultaneously is fundamental. Indeed, it may turn out that behavioral data can provide us with better answers to questions about the time course of processing than it can on questions of mental representation or underlying computational architecture.

At a more substantive level, one of the main themes to emerge from the research surveyed above is the idea that the effects of mental sets are more pervasive than had previously been thought. As described in the first sections of this chapter, a variety of proposals for "wired-in" attention capture by particular stimulus attributes have been effectively challenged; attention, it turns out, is subject to a far greater degree of top-down control than was suspected 10 years ago. A second broad conclusion is that the effects of practice appear much more circumscribed than was previously appreciated. Although it may turn out that some mental operations are truly subject to automatization in the strongest sense, it appears quite unlikely that this holds nearly as broadly as was once suspected.

More recently a symbolic and connectionist model (CAP2) has been proposed (Schneider & Chein, 2003). The authors describe a computational model of human performance in the controlled and automatic process modes, which also explains the transitions between the modes.

The CAP2 model seeks to account for the phenomena of automatic processing, and to explain the role of controlled processing in a wide range of cognitive tasks.

Conceptually, CAP2 is a hybrid cognitive architecture, incorporating both symbolic (e.g., ACT-R) and connectionist (e.g., PDP) elements. In actuality, the CAP2 architecture is implemented with entirely connectionist components, but has networks that operate as sequential control structures that can configure the network to behave as a production system (e.g., to implement condition–action rules with variable binding-based operations). The hybrid architecture is intended to capitalize on the complementary strengths exhibited by the two modelling approaches, as they relate to controlled and automatic processing. Specifically, production system architectures account well for symbolic variable binding behaviors, in which an algorithm in memory takes on a specific, yet arbitrary, input as the value of one of its variables (e.g., in VM search, an incoming stimulus is mapped to a variable representing the trial input, and then the particular form of the stimulus is compared to internal representations of the target stimuli). Symbolic architectures can easily perform such variable binding tasks for arbitrary symbols (e.g., determine whether the following sequence is a palindrome of letters, "tzppzt"), while it is very difficult to build connectionist architectures that perform such tasks without extended training of the stimuli.

Symbolic processing has the disadvantage of producing representations that are often brittle and exhibit limited transfer. Connectionist processes, in contrast, show good generalization and parallel processing, but often at the cost of very long learning times (tens of thousands of trials), and an inability to transfer to analogous tasks that do not include similar stimulus elements. These properties of symbolic and connectionist architectures can be mapped onto the relative advantages of controlled and automatic processing. Recall that automatic processes operate through a relatively permanent set of associative connections and require an appreciable amount of consistent training to develop fully. Automatic processes therefore behave much like most connectionist networks (after they have been trained). In contrast, a controlled process "may be set up, altered, and applied in novel situations for which automatic sequences have never been learned" [7]. Accordingly, controlled processing proceeds similarly to processing in most production system architectures.

The model of Schneider and Chein [42] enables predictions at the micro level (type of units), macro level (organizational structure of cortical connections), and process levels (nature of executive function). Providing a biologically feasible model for human cognition requires a detailing of a comprehensive architecture. It is a challenge to relate the multiple modes of human cognition to the rich complexity of brain structure. Most models based on neural principles seek to demonstrate the ability of parsimonious architectural elements to predict human behavioral performance (e.g., computation by populations of additive connectionist units, as in McClelland & Rumelhart, [43]). In contrast, the modules in CAP2 attempt to capture the computational richness of the diverse neuronal assemblies that comprise cortical modular columns (hypercolumns), which are found to recur throughout the cortex with regionally specialized connection patterns [44, 45, 46, 47].

One of our goals in developing the CAP2 model has been to implement symbolic and connectionist processing through the use of a modular connectionist architecture and to provide explicit quantitative representations of both the development of automaticity and the nature of controlled processing. The model achieves this goal by employing a Control System that monitors and modulates activity in a large Data Matrix of connectionist modules. The connectionist modules in CAP2 are intended to mimic the modular quality of cortical structure.

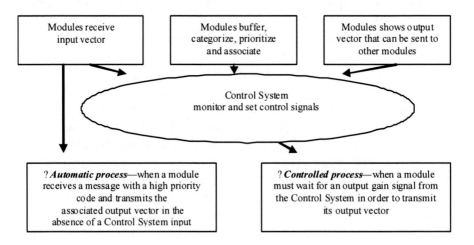

Figure 17. The Schneider and Chein's model

The model of Schneider and Chein [42] start with the consideration that the brain is composed of many modules. Each of the modules in CAP2 can receive input vectors, and can locally buffer, categorize, prioritize and associate (learn) an output vector that can be sent to other modules. The Control System is implemented as a set of interlinked connectionist processors (with properties resembling a symbolic architecture) that monitor and set control signals sent to the network of connectionist modules. These control signals alter functional connectivity within the architecture, thereby enabling a wide variety of cognitive operations.

## CONCLUSION

In this chapter automatic and controlled processes were analized. Schneider and Shiffrin distinguished between automatic and controlled processes and showed that some automatic processes develop with practice. However, they do not fully explain *how* this happens.

Another approach seems to underline that there is no clear distinction but a gradation between the two processes [17]. Gopher seeks evidence to support the idea that attention management is a skill and that it can be learnt through training. He argues that we would need to show: first, that subjects do actually have the potential to control their allocation of attention: second, that this potential is not always fulfilled, in so far as subjects may fail to maintain control: and last, that with appropriate training, difficulties of control can be overcome.

Since the criteria for automatic processes are rarely satisfied in practice. Norman and Shallice developed the schema activation model in which they propose two control systems (contention scheduling and SAS), distinguishing between fully automatic and partially automatic processes, which is consistent with the finding that relatively few processes satisfy the criteria for automaticity.

Critics to the models of dyadic processes come from different views: it is not evident that automatic processing is free of attentional limitations [50, 51], there are attentional limitations in tasks that are thought to be performed automatically [52, 53, 54], many resources other than attention may limit performance [55], automatization may not reflect the gradual withdrawal of attention [56]. Another critical stance comes from Pashler who thinks that it is certainly the case that serial and parallel models may mimic each other in certain contexts, and that the phenomenon of involuntary attention capture, often presumed to be entirely bottom-up and stimulus driven, turns out to be subtly influenced by top-down goals. He shows also that attention capture, a phenomenon that appears at first glance to be entirely under top-down cognitive control, turns out to be heavily influenced by bottom-up, stimulus-driven processing.

The Instance Theory of automatization [2], is an alternative view to these conceptualizations. Logan [2] assumes that each time we solve the problem we get a new instance of the problem stored in memory. Logan's model is self-terminating and parallel. This means that we are both trying to work out the solution the long way and retrieve it from memory at the same time. As soon as we determine a solution (whichever way you do it) we stop working on the problem. Skills become increasingly automatic as more and more instances are added to memory and it becomes increasingly likely that the problem will be solved by memory. In the same way, Logan's model says that when solving a problem we both try to craft a solution and at the same time look for an old solution in memory. And then we stop as soon as either method provides a solution. The more old solutions there are in memory, the more needles there are in the haystack, the more likely we are to solve the problem through memory and the faster we should be able to solve the problem.

Schneider and Chein [42] assume on the other hand that dual processing theory has seen very productive development in the last 25 years. The authors have described a computational model of human performance in the controlled and automatic process modes, which also explains the transitions between the modes. The modeling work has led to an understanding of the relevant processing tradeoffs, and to elaboration of the expected computational architecture. A rapidly advancing brain imaging literature provides a forum for tests of this model, and offers initial support for key concepts in dual processing theory. The physiology has also stimulated the implementation of new concepts in the model, such as the presence of inner loop communications and declarative memory coding of inner loop information.

## REFERENCES

[1]    Anderson, J.R. (1983). *The architecture of cognition.* Cambridge, MA: Harvard University Press.
[2]    Logan, G. D. (1988). Toward an instance theory of automatization.. *Psychological Review, 95*, 492-527.
[3]    Pashler, H., Johnston, J., & Ruthruff, E. (2001). Attention and Performance. *Annual Review of Psychology, 52*, 629-651.

[4]     Stanovich, K.E. (1987). The impact of automaticity theory. *Journal of learning disabilities, 20, 3,* 167-168.

[5]     Neely, J. H. (1977). Semantic priming and retrieval from lexical memory: Roles of inhibition less spreading activation and limited-capacity attention. *Journal of Experimental Ps.\'chologv: General, 106,* 226-254.

[6]     Posner, M.I., & Snyder, C.R.R. (1975). Attention and cognitive control. In R. Solso (ed.), *Information Processing and Cognition: The Loyola Symposium.* Hillsdale, N.J.: Lawrence Erlbaum Associates.

[7]     Schneider, W.. & Shiffrin. R.M. (1977). Controlled and automatic human information processing: LDetection. search and attention. *Psychological Review, 84,* 1-66.

[8]     Zbrodoff, N. J., & Logan, G. D. (1986). On the autonomy of mental processes: A case study of arithmetic. *Journal of Experimental Psychology: General, 115,2,* 118–130.

[9]     McLeod, P., McLaughlin, C., & Nimmo-Smith, I. (1986). Information encapsulation and automaticity: Evidence from the visual control of finely timed actions. In M. I. Posner & O. S. M. Marin(Eds.), *Attention and performance XI* (pp. 391–406). Hillsdale,NJ: Erlbaum

[10]   Carr, T.H., McCauley, C., Sperber, R.D., & Parmalee, C.M. (1982). Words , pictures, and priming: On semantic activation, conscious identification, and the automaticity of information processing. *Journal of Experimental Psychology: Human Perception and Performance, 8,* 757-777.

[11]   Norman, D.A. & Shallice, T. (1986). Attention to action: Willed and automatic control of behaviour. In R. Davison, G. Shwartz & D. Shapiro (Eds.). *Consciousness and self regulation: Advances in research and theory.* New York: Plenum.

[12]   Posner, M.I. (1978). *Chronometric explorations of mind.* Hillsdale. NJ: Lawrence Erlbaum Associates Inc.

[13]   Treisman, A., Vieira, A., & Hayes, A. (1992). Automatic and preattentive processing. *American Journal of Psychology, 105, 341-362.*

[14]   Spelke, E.S. & Tsivkin, S. (2001). Language and number: A bilingual training study. *Cognition, 78,* 45–88.

[15]   Umilta' C., Moscovitch M. (1994). Attention and performance XV: Conscious and nonconscious information processing. Cambridge: MIT Press.

[16]   Neuman, O. (1984). Automatic processing: A review of recent findings and a plea for an old theory. InW.Printz & Sanders, A. (Eds.). *Cognition and motor processes.* Berlin: Springer.

[17] Carr, T.H. (1992). Automaticity and Cognitive Anatomy: Is Word Recognition "Automatic? . *The American Journal of Psychology*, *105*, *2*, 201-237.

[18] Bargh, J. A. (1989). Conditional automaticity: Varieties of automatic influences in social perception and cognition. In J. S. Uleman & J. A. Bargh (Eds.), *Unintended Thought* (pp. 3–51).New York, NY: Guilford Press.

[19] Tzelgov, J. (1997). Specifying the relations between automaticity and consciousness: A theoretical note. *Consciousness and Cognition, 6*, 441-451.

[20] Palmeri,T.J. (1997). Exemplan similarity and the development of automaticity. *Journal of experimental psychology: Learning, Memory and Cognition, 23* , 324-354.

[21] Rickard, T. C. (1997). Bending the power law: A CMPL theory of strategy shifts and the automatization of cognitive skills. *Journal of Experimental Psychology: General, 126*, 288–311.

[22] Vallacher, R., & Wegner, D. (1987). What do people think they are doing? Action identification and human behavior. *Psychological Review, 94*, 3-15

[23] Jacoby, L. (1991). A process discrimination framework: Separating automatic from intentional uses of memory. *Journal of Memory and Language, 30*, 531-541.

[24] Saling, L.L., & Phillips, J.G. (2007). Automatic behaviour: Efficient not mindless. *Brain Research Bulletin, 73*, 1-20.

[25] Pashler, H.(2001). Involuntary orienting to flashing distracters in delayed search. In C.L. Folk & B. Gibson(Eds). *Attraction, distraction and action : multiple perspectives on attentional capture. Advances in psychology.* Elsevier.

[26] Posner, M.I. (1980). Orienting of attention. *Quarterly Journal of Experimental Psychology, 32*, 3-25.

[27] Atkinson, R.C. & Shiffrin, R.M. (1968). Human memory: A proposed system and controlprocesses. In K.W.Spence & J.D.Spence (Eds.), *The psychology of learning and motivation(Vol.2).* New York: Academic Press.

[28] Styles, E. A. (2007). *The psychology of attention.* London: The Taylor & Francis e-Library.

[29] Logan, G. D. (1979). On the use of a concurrent memory load to measure attention and automaticity. *Journal of Experimental Psychology: Human Perception and Performance, 5*, 189-207.

[30] Boronat, C.B.,& Logan, G.D. (2005) The role of attention in automatization: does attention operate at encoding, or retrieval, or both? *Mem Cognit.; 25*, 1, 36-46.

[31] Treisman, A. (1992). Perceiving and not perceiving objects. *American psychologist, 47*,862-875.

[32] Treisman, A., Vieira, A., & Hayes, A. (1992). Automatic and preattentive processing. *American Journal of Psychology, 105, 341-362.*

[33] McClelland, J.L.. & Rumelhart, D.E. (1981). An interactive activation model of context effects in letter perception: Part 1. An account of basic findings. *Psychological Review, 85,* 375-407.

[34] Baddeley, A.D. (1986). *Working memory.* Oxford: Oxford University Press.

[35] Shallice, T. & Burgess, P.W. (1993). Supervisory control of action and thought selection. In A.D.Baddeley & L. Weiskrantz (Eds.), *Attention: Awareness, selection, and control.* Oxford: Oxford University Press.

[36] Shallice, T. Burgess, P., Schon, F. & Baxter, D. (1989). The origins of utilization behaviour. *Brain, 112,* 1587-1598.

[37] Broadbent, D.E. (1984). The Maltese Cross: A new simplistic model for memory. *Behavioural and Brain Sciences, 7,* 55—68.

[38] Yantis, S. & Johnston, J.C. (1990). On the locus of visual selection: Evidence from focused attention tasks. *Journal of Experimental Psychology: Human Perception and Performance, 16*,135-149.

[39] Theeuwes, Y. (1991). Cross-dimensional perceptual selectivity. *Perception end psychophysics, 50,* 184-193.

[40] Townshend, J. M. & Duka, T. (2001). Attentional bias associated with alcohol cues: differences between heavy and occasional social drinkers. *Psychopharmacology*,157,1, 67–74.

[41] Schneider, W., & Chein, J.M. (2003) . Controlled & automatic processing: behavior, theory, and biological mechanisms. *Cognitive Science,* 27, 525-559.

[42] McClelland. J.L.. & Rumelhart. D.E. (1981). An interactive activation model of context effects in letter perception: Part 1. An account of basic findings. *Psychological Review, 85,* 375-407.

[43] Felleman , D.Y & Van Essen, D.C. (1991). Distributed hierarchical processing in primate cerebral contex. *Cerebral contex, 1,* 1-47.

[44] Goodman, P. H., Courtenay Wilson, E., Maciokas, J. B., Harris, F. C., Gupta, A. G., Louis, J. L., Markram, H. (2001). *Large-scale parallel simulation of physiologically realistic multicolumn sensory cortex NIPS.*

[45] Martin, K. A. (1988). The Wellcome Prize lecture. From single cells to simple circuits in the cerebral cortex. *Quarterly Journal of Experimental Physiology,* 73(5), 637–702.

[46] White, E. L. (1989). *Cortical circuits synaptic organization of the cerebral cortex. Structure, function and Theory.* Boston: Birkhauser.

[47] Allport, D.A. (1980). Patterns and actions.In G.Claxton (Ed.), *Cognitive psychology: New directions.* London: Routledge & Kegan Paul.

[48] Allport, D.A. (1988). What concept of consciousness? In A.J.Marcel & E. Bisiach (Eds.),*Consciousness in contemporary science.* Oxford: Oxford University Press.

[49] Cheng, P.W. (1985). Restructuring versus automaticity: alternative accounts of skill acquisition. *Psychological review, 92, 33,* 414-423.

[50] Ryan, C. (1983) Reassessing the automaticity-control distinction: Item recognition as a paradigm case. *Psychological Review, 90, 2.*

[51] Kahneman. D., & Chajczyk. D. (1983). Tests of the automaticity of reading: Dilution of Stroop effects by colour-irrelevant stimuli. *Journal of Experimental Psychology*: Human Perception and Performance, 9, 497—509.

[52] Paap, K.R., Ogden, W.C. (1981). Letter encoding is an obligatory but capacity-demanding operation. *Journal of Experimental Psychology: Human Perception and Performance, 7, 3,* 518-527

[53] Regan, J. (1981). Automaticity and learning: Effect of familiarity on naming letters. *Journal of Experimental Psychology: Human Perception and Performance, 7,* 180-195.

[54] Wickens, C.D. (1984). Processing resources in attention. In R. Parsuramaii & D.R. Davies (Eds.), *Varieties of attention.* Orlando. FL: Academic Press.

[55] Hirst, W.. Spelke. E.S.. Reeves. C. Caharack. G.. & Neisser, U. (1980). Dividing attention without alternation or automaticity. *Journal of Experimental Psychology: General, 109,* 98-117.

# Chapter 2

# PARADIGMS OF INVESTIGASTION OF AUTOMATIC AND CONTROLLED PROCESSES

## ABSTRACT

The purpose of this chapter is to present some methodologies that investigate the process of automatization through different paradigms. Initially the search paradigm that is the major empirical paradigm in which automatic and controlled processes are explored is presented; afterwards the Stroop task and the priming paradigm are presented. With the Stroop paradigm we are able to discover that automaticity is influenced by task demand: word reading in adults is an extremely well-learned skill, but in early readers, the effect is not present, or may even be reversed. In the priming paradigm, where the basic design of the experiment is to precede the target stimulus by a neutral warning signal, results showed that when the prime was a poor predictor of the target there was benefit but no cost. When the prime was of high validity the benefit accrued more rapidly than the cost. This effect was interpreted as showing that the allocation of conscious attention takes more time than automatic activation. Then the Merrill procedure with a visual search paradigm is analyzed and finally the clock test of Moron is presented. The Visual search paradigm allows us to manipulate content (e.g. physical and semantic identity) and is mainly linked to the underlying logic of automatized processes implied by learning. The logic of the repeated visual search paradigm is linked to automatized processes implied by learning: automatization typically develops when the same stimuli have to be detected consistently over many trials. In the concluding section some thoughts about the relationship between different paradigms are offered.

## THE SEARCH PARADIGM

The major empirical paradigm in which automatic and controlled processes are explored is the search paradigm. Figure 1 illustrates the search paradigm [1].

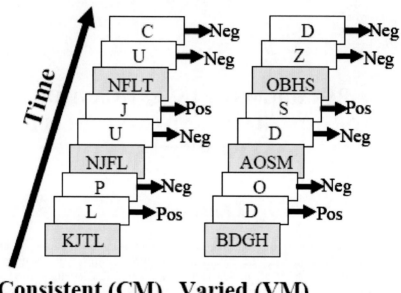

## Consistent (CM)  Varied (VM)

## Mapping

Figure 1. Visual search task

CM and VM refer to the consistency manipulation. The subject is given a memory set of typically one to five items that they must remember. Then the subject sees a set of sequentially (single-channel) or simultaneously (multiple channel) presented probe items that he or she must search through. If any of the probe items matches any of the items in memory, a target is detected, and the subject makes a positive response. When a probe item does not match any of the memory set items, it is referred to as a distractor, and the subject makes a negative response or no response at all. For example, the subject may be given a memory set of the letters "KJTL" to remember, and then a probe (e.g., "L" or "P"). The subject compares each memory set item to the probe item, looking for a match. In VM, items can be a target on one trial, but then become a distractor on the next trial. Therefore, if the task has a varied mapping, then a given stimulus may require varied responses from trial to trial. In contrast, in CM, items that have been targets on one trial never become distractors in subsequent trials. Therefore, if the task has a consistent mapping, then a given stimulus always requires the same response.

With reference to automatic and controlled processes, extended consistent training is required in order to develop automatic processing, while controlled processes can be established in a few trials and under varied mapping situations. As mentioned above, automatic search training develops after extended consistent search.

For automatic search in detection experiments, the rate and effectiveness of learning are a function of the degree of consistency [2]. Shiffrin & Schneider [3] showed, as we see above in the first chapter, that it is specifically the consistent mapping, rather than learning to categorize items rapidly (category search), that is critical for automaticity. Subjects began the experiment under varied mapping conditions in which they learned that letters belonged to one of two categories (GMFP vs. CNHD), but the category being searched for was varied from trial to trial (e.g., on one trial they searched for the letters GMFP with distractors CNHD, and on the next trial they searched for the opposite set of CNHD with distractors GMFP). The category training continued for 25 sessions until the memory set size effect for searching for 2 versus 4 members of the category was the same, and performance was at asymptote. At this point, the search was made consistent, with one category being always the target. There was a dramatic improvement in processing speed, and a reduction in effort at the point where consistent search was introduced. This result supports the view that automaticity, and the automatic attention response, emerges only when the stimulus-response mappings remain consistent. It is important to further note that the consistency of training need not be at the exemplar level.

# THE STROOP TASK

In the Stroop [4] task (figure 2), participants have to identify the colors in which color words and control stimuli are visually displayed (for a review, see MacLeod [5]).

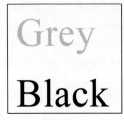            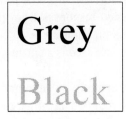

Congruent ink color               Incongruent ink color

Figure. 2 Stimuli of Stroop paradigm

Another example is having to count the number of characters present in a display, when the characters themselves are digits (see figure 3).

$$2\ 4\ 7\ 1\ 3$$

Figure. 3 Digits stimuli of Stroop paradigm

Jacoby, Lindsay and Hessels [6] point out that usually the Stroop effect is asymmetrical: in the case of colour words written in an incongruent ink colour, the word interferes with the ink naming, but not vice versa.

It seems that the word automatically activates its response and although conscious control can prevent the response from being made overtly, there is a time cost while the intended response, ink naming, gains control of overt action. The asymmetry arises because the ink naming is less strongly mapped onto a response and is easily overcome by the stronger mapping of the word to its response [6]. Word reading in adults is an extremely well-learned skill, but in early readers, the effect is not present, or may even be reversed. On the other hand, the direction of interference may depend on task demands: when the task involves deciding whether stimuli match physically, judgements are made more quickly for colours than words, and in this case, experiments show that there is more interference from colours on words [7]. However, if the ink colour and word are congruent the word may facilitate vocal colour naming [8].

Posner and Snyder [9] suggest that there is automatic parallel processing of both features of the stimulus until close to output. Automatic processing cannot be prevented, but conscious attention can be used flexibly. So, while some cognitive operations proceed automatically- others take place under strategic, conscious, attentional control which is deployed according to the subject's intentions.

## THE PRIMING PARADIGM

To analyze automatic and controlled processes, Posner and Snyder [9] used a prime paradigm. On each trial the subject was presented with a priming stimulus, either a letter or a plus sign (figure 4).

Prime                          Prime

Figure 4. Stimuli of the priming paradigm

The prime was followed by a pair of letters and the task was to decide, as quickly as possible, whether the letters were the same or different. There were two basic predictions. First, the prime would automatically activate its representation in memory, so that if the prime was A and the pair of letters to be matched were AA, response would be facilitated because the activation in memory was confirmed. According to the view of Posner and Snyder [9], if the prime was different from the target, there would be no inhibition produced by this automatic memory activation on other responses.

The basic design of the experiment is to precede the target stimulus by either a neutral warning signal, in this case the plus sign, or a non-neutral prime which should, if attended, bias target processing. The probability that the prime would be a valid cue for the target was manipulated, as it was assumed that the subjects would adopt a strategy whereby they invested more or less attention in the prime depending on whether or not they thought it would be a valid predictor of the target. According to the theory, when the subject pays little processing capacity to the prime, a valid cue will automatically produce facilitation but no costs. However, when the subject "actively attends" to the prime there will be facilitatory benefits from both automatic activation and from conscious attention if the prime is valid, but when the prime is not valid there will be inhibitory costs due to strategic processing.

Results showed that when the prime was a poor predictor of the target there was benefit but no cost. When the prime was of high validity the benefit accrues more rapidly than the cost. This effect was interpreted as showing that the allocation of conscious attention takes more time than automatic activation. The differential time course of facilitatory and inhibitory effects suggested a real difference between the two kinds of processing.

## THE SEMANTIC PRIMING PARADIGM

Kiefer [10] underlines that semantic priming paradigm is a good paradigm to investigate automatic semantic processes. During the last decades, convincing evidence has been accumulated that the semantic meaning of masked words that cannot be consciously identified is activated and can influence processing of subsequently presented stimuli [10]. While it is well accepted that unconsciously perceived masked stimuli can prime an associated motor response (response priming; see Klotz & Neumann, [12; 13], it has been questioned that unconsciously perceived masked stimuli are processed also at the level of semantic meaning [13, 14]. However, a variety of studies using the semantic priming paradigm, which is not compromised by confounding response priming effects, have reliably shown that semantic meaning is extracted from unconsciously perceived stimuli [10, 15, 16, 17] for semantic priming during the attentional blink, see Rolke, Heil, Streb, & Henninghausen, [18]).

Complementary to response priming, the masked semantic priming paradigm is a powerful tool to study the nature of unconscious perception and to study the modulatory effects on automatic processes.

In the masked semantic priming procedure, conscious perception of the prime is eliminated by displaying a pattern mask (e.g., a random sequence of letters) before and after the prime.

Unconscious semantic activation is demonstrated when the masked prime word facilitates the processing of the target stimulus. Semantic priming has been frequently observed in lexical decision tasks in which subjects have to decide whether a target word (e.g., "lemon") is a real word or a pseudoword. Reactions are faster and more accurate if a semantically related prime word (e.g., "sour") precedes the target in comparison to a condition in which an unrelated word (e.g., "house") precedes the target.

Two general cognitive mechanisms have been proposed to underlie semantic priming effects: Firstly, unconscious automatic spreading of activation and secondly, conscious strategic semantic processing [9]. According to the first cognitive mechanism, semantic priming reflects the automatic spread of activation in semantic networks. The presentation of a prime stimulus is thought to activate the corresponding conceptual representation in a semantic network, and activation spreads to semantically related nodes, hereby increasing their activation level. Hence, if a word denoting a related concept is presented, its recognition is facilitated. According to Posner and Snyder [9] automatic spread of activation does not depend on capacity-limited attentional processes. In contrast, according to the second class of cognitive mechanisms (strategic semantic processing), semantic priming is the result of controlled attentional processes such as semantic matching or semantic expectation (for an overview, see Neely, [19]).

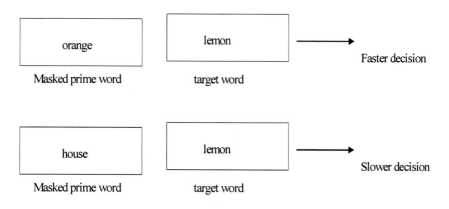

Figure 5. Stimuli of the masked semantic priming procedure

## VISUAL SEARCH PARADIGM - MERRIL PROCEDURE

Using the Merril [20] procedure automatic and effortful processes can be investigated. This procedure involves an integration of the codification methodology and the memory load methodology.

To inquire the codification processes, classic methodology uses pairs of pictures. Subjects are instructed to identify, as quickly as possible, when two stimuli are identical (physical identity, figure 5) or when two stimuli belong to the same category (categorical identity, figure 6).

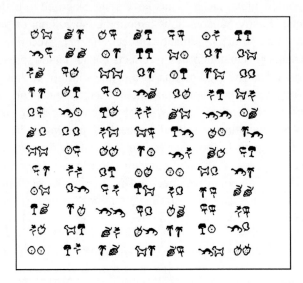

Figure 6. Physical identity stimuli of visual search paradigm

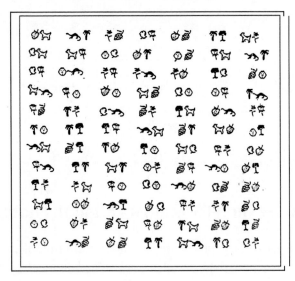

Figure 7. Categorical identity stimuli of visual search paradigm

The visual information processing task used in some experiments are variations on the tasks described by Melnik and Das [21], involving judgment of physical identity and semantic identity of pairs of pictures (see figures). The pictures consisted of fruits (strawberries and grapes), flowers (roses and daisies), trees (palms and elm trees), faces (in frontal and profile view) and animals (dinosaurs and dogs).

In the Merril procedure classic methodology is combined with a memory load task. Subjects have to repeat a list of numbers during the codification task. Memory load is manipulated by increasing or decreasing the memory set size. The purpose is to measure the level of cognitive load that interferes with performance.

The underlying logic of this procedure is that the automatism of the coding process could be identified by examining the difference between coding speed and identification accuracy of the stimuli (Dulaney & Ellis, 1994; Logan, Taylor & Etherthon, 1996) using the two procedures: the physical and semantic identification procedure (Melnik and Das, 1992; Fabio e Cossutta, 2001) and the integrated procedure of Merrill (1992).

Since automatic processes can be accomplished simultaneously with other cognitive processes without interference (Hasher & Zacks, 1979; Posner & Snyder, 1975; Lavie, 1995), any difference in interference of memory load could reflect a difference in automatic performance. The rationale is that if subjects are able to perform the selection tasks equally well, both in the presence and in the absence of a memory load, then one can suppose that the selection is automatic; if, on the contrary, the subjects show a penalization due to the memory interference, then one can suppose that the selection is not automatic.

With regard to physical and semantic identity [21, 22] the assumption is that when the selective attention is directed towards the physical characteristics of the stimulus, the subject has to simply recognise the physical identity and fewer semantic resources. Under these circumstances, automatic processes can be applied.

When the selective attention shifts to the semantic characteristics of the stimulus, the subject has to recognize the individual items, identify their category and employ semantic resources. In this latter case, conciously controlled and directed coding processes are necessary.

Merril [20] used this integrated procedure with both mentally retarded and normal participants. His data show that both are subjected to a cost in coding in the presence of a mnestic load. Therefore his data indicate little about the lack of automaticity in subjects with mental retardation. To explain these data Merril [20] talks about *partially automated* coding processes that are those processes which can be performed without attentional resources but, nevertheless, benefit from additional resources in terms of speed and accuracy.

## REPEATED VISUAL SEARCH PARADIGM

Automatization typically develops when the same stimuli have to be detected consistently over many trials.

Szymura, Slabosz and Orzechowski [23] used the Clock Test to study the automatization process[24]. The Clock Test consists of 40 target signals and 40 distracting dials among stimuli (figure 7). Subjects had to detect the stimulus (an icon) representing hours on the clock (the dial). Other icons served as noise. The icon of 4 o'clock was the target to detect. Subjects had 2 minutes to complete the test. They had to repeat the same task for three times (figure 8).

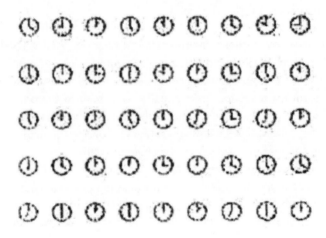

Figure 8. Stimuli of the clock test

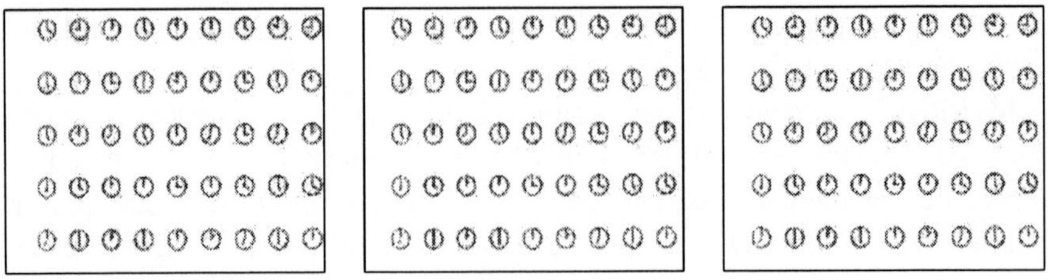

Figure 9. The same task presented for three times

The index of automatization is calculated by the difference in correctness of selectivity mechanism between the third and the first trial and the difference in the number of errors between the third and the first trial.

Normally the three measures of task performance that are recorded are:

-   the number of scanned stimuli – SPEED ( in a period of 2 minutes of continuous attention);
-   the number of false alarms – FA (erroneous "detection");
-   the number of omissions – OM (lack of detection).

The stimuli in repeated search paradigm can be varied. In another work [25] the "d2" attention test, repeated for three times, was used to measure the intensity of automatization [26]. Also in this case the number of scanned stimuli, the number of false alarms and the number of omissions were calculated.

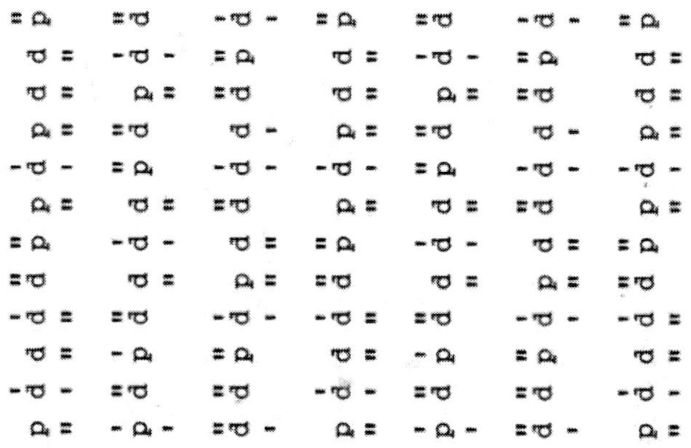

Figure 10. Stimuli of "d2" attention test

# GO/NO-GO PARADIGM

Despite the fact that the go/no-go paradigm and the stop-signal paradigms normally refer to the literature that investigates response inhibition, Verbruggen and Logan [1] present a possible way to apply them to enhance automatic and controlled processes.

In the go/no-go paradigm, subjects are presented with a series of stimuli and are told to respond when a go stimulus is presented and to withhold their response when a no-go stimulus is presented (e.g., press the response key for the letter K but do not press the response key for the letter L, figure 9).

The mapping of stimuli onto go and no-go responses is explained at the beginning of the experiment and typically remains the same throughout the experiment. In this paradigm, the index of inhibitory control is the probability of executing a response on a no-go trial [p(respond|no-go)].

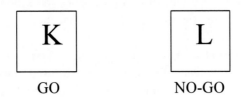

GO                              NO-GO

Figure 11. Stimuli of the so/no go paradigm

## STOP-SIGNAL PARADIGM

In the stop-signal paradigm, subjects usually perform a choice reaction task on no-stop-signal trials (e.g., press the left response key for the letter K and press the right response key for the letter L). On a random selection of the trials (stop-signal trials), a stop signal is presented after a variable delay (stop-signal delay or SSD), which instructs subjects to withhold the response to the go stimulus on those trials. The first index of inhibitory control is the probability of responding on stop-signal trials [p(respond|signal)], which is often evaluated as a function of SSD. The second index of inhibitory control is an estimate of the covert latency of the stop process, stop-signal reaction time (SSRT).

The go/no-go and stop-signal paradigms are very common tools in the literature that investigates response inhibition in basic research in cognitive science and cognitive neuroscience.

As Verbruggen and Logan [1] underline, both paradigms have been used to study response-inhibition deficits in clinical populations such as children and adults with attention-deficit/hyperactivity disorder [27, 28, 29, 30]. In addition, researchers have used the paradigms to study effects of aging and development [31, 32, 33, 34] and to test individual differences in constructs such as impulsivity [35, 36].

In the response-inhibition literature, it is common to generalize the results obtained in the go/no-go paradigm to the stop-signal paradigm, and vice versa. The rationale is that response inhibition in the two paradigms is achieved in the same way.

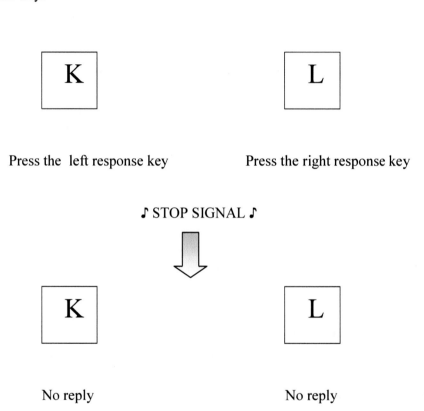

Figure 12. Stimuli of the stop signal paradigm

Performance in both paradigms is typically described in terms of a race between two competing processes: a *go process* and a *stop process* [37, 38]. In the go/no-go paradigm, the go process is triggered by stimulus presentation because of a prepotent response tendency, and the stop process is triggered by the identification of the no-go stimulus. In the stop-signal paradigm, the go process is triggered by the presentation of the go stimulus and the stop process is triggered by the presentation of the stop signal. The probability of responding on a no-go trial or a stopsignal trial depends on the relative finishing time of the go process and the stop process.

When the stop process finishes before the go process, response inhibition is successful and no response is emitted; when the go processes finishes before the stop process, response inhibition is unsuccessful and the response is incorrectly emitted.

Verbruggen and Logan [1] used these paradigms in a different manner. They investigated whether activating the stop goal in the go/no-go paradigm is an executively controlled process. More specifically, the authors investigated whether the stop goal can be automatically activated through memory retrieval of consistent associations between the no-go stimulus and stopping. Results show that response inhibition can be achieved through either automatic or controlled processing, depending on the consistency of associations between stimuli and stopping.

## STEM-COMPLETION TEST

To disentangle the contributions of automatic and controlled processes, Debner and Jacoby [39] and Meier, Morger and Graf [40] examined stem-completion test performance in a condition that required subjects not to give as stem-completions any primes they were able to identify and remember [41, 42]. See figure 11 for an example of the procedure.

As illustrated in figure 11, each trial started with a fixation point, a plus sign that was displayed for 500 ms. The fixation point was replaced by a 200-ms blank interval, which in turn was replaced by a 200-ms mask consisting of a random series of letters (i.e., EMXDGF), then by the display of a prime, another 200-ms random letter-mask and finally a word-stem. The display duration of the primes, which varied according to conditions, was 0, 16, 33, 50, or 66 ms, respectively. In the 0-ms prime condition, a 16-ms blank was inserted between the two masks. As depicted in Figure 1, in the delayed-stems condition, a blank was displayed for 2 s immediately before each word-stem. In all conditions, the word-stem remained on the screen until the subject entered a completion via the keyboard or until 15 s had elapsed. Then the next trial began. Subjects were instructed to complete each word-stem with the first five- or six letter word that came to mind. They responded by entering these completions on the keyboard. In addition, they were instructed to report any prime word they were able to identify and not use this word as a stem completion. In the delayed-stems condition, subjects were also informed that a 2-s blank would be shown immediately before each word-stem. Furthermore, they were advised to report any identified primes either during this blank period or after completing the word-stem. The experimenter recorded immediately all prime words reported by subjects.

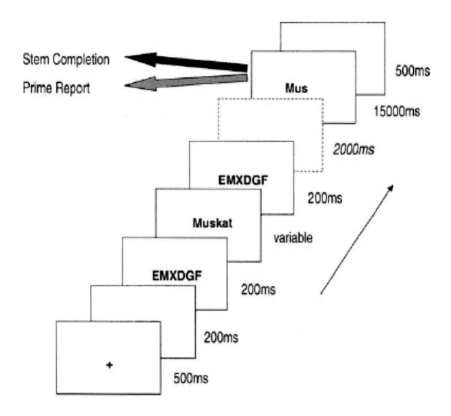

Figure 13. The figure shows the sequence of events that occurred on each trial. The solid displays represent the events in the immediate-stems condition, and the dashed display shows the addition of the blank in the delayed-stems condition.

The main part of the experiment consisted of two blocks of 70 trials, with five letter words serving as primes for one block and six-letter words for the other. The order of the blocks was counterbalanced across subjects. The two blocks were separated by a brief pause.

In the work of Debner and Jacoby [39] masked primes were showed either for 50 ms or for 500 ms, and the stem-completion test results showed a priming effect in the short-display condition but not in the long-display condition. Debner and Jacoby interpreted this pattern of results as evidence that the short displays were sufficient to facilitate the subsequent automatic reprocessing of the prime words, but not long enough to permit their consciously controlled processing. Thus, when instructed not to give as completions any words that had appeared as primes, subjects produced the prime words as completions only in the short-display condition where their production was facilitated by automatic processes. By contrast, in the long-display condition, subjects were able to rely on controlled processes and thus avoided giving the primes as stem completions. The interpretations offered by Debner and Jacoby [39] and by Merikle et al. [43] focus on the widespread assumption that automatic processes are faster than controlled processes. By this assumption, it follows that the former but not the latter would influence performance when prime-words are displayed for only a brief duration.

## CONCLUSION

In this chapter some paradigms of automatic and controlled processes were analyzed. Existing procedures are many. They allow us to focus on different facetings of automatic and controlled processes.

In the search paradigm it is shown that for automatic search in detection experiments, the rate and effectiveness of learning is a function of the degree of consistency [3]. Shiffrin & Schneider [2] showed that it is specifically the consistent mapping, rather than learning to categorize items rapidly (category search), that is critical for automaticity.

With the Stroop paradigm we are able to discover that automaticity is influenced by task demand: word reading in adults is an extremely well-learned skill, but in early readers, the effect is not present, or may even be reversed.

In the priming paradigm, where the basic design of the experiment is to precede the target stimulus by either a neutral warning signal, in this case the plus sign, or a non-neutral prime which should, if attended, bias target processing. Results showed that when the prime was a poor predictor of the target there was benefit but no cost. When the prime was of high validity the benefit accrues more rapidly than the cost. This effect was interpreted as showing that the allocation of conscious attention takes more time than automatic activation.

Kiefer [10] underlines that the semantic priming paradigm is a good paradigm to investigate automatic semantic processes. Semantic priming has been frequently observed in lexical decision tasks in which subjects have to decide whether a target word (e.g., "lemon") is a real word or a pseudoword. Reactions, as we see above, are faster and more accurate if a semantically related prime word (e.g., "sour") precedes the target in comparison to a condition in which an unrelated word (e.g., "house") precedes the target. Also in the masked semantic priming procedure, conscious perception of the prime is eliminated by displaying a pattern mask (e.g., a random sequence of letters) before and after the prime and unconscious semantic activation is demonstrated when the masked prime word facilitates the processing of the target stimulus.

The Visual search paradigm, allows us to manipulate content (e.g. physical and semantic identity) and is mainly linked to the underlying logic of automatized processes implied by learning: since automatic processes can be accomplished simultaneously with other cognitive processes without interference [44, 9, 45], any difference in interference of memory load could reflect a difference in automatic performance. The rationale is that if subjects are able to perform the selection tasks equally well, both in the presence and in the absence of a memory load, then one can suppose that the selection is automatic; if, on the contrary, the subjects show a penalization due to the memory interference, then one can suppose that the selection is not automatic.

Also the logic of the repeated visual search paradigm is linked to automatized processes implied by learning: automatization typically develops when the same stimuli has to be detected consistently over many trials. The index of automatization in this case was calculated by the difference in correctness of selectivity mechanism between the third and the first trial and the difference in the number of errors between the third and the first trial.

Despite the go/no-go paradigm and the stop-signal paradigms normally refer to the literature that investigate response inhibition, Verbruggen and Logan [1] present a possible way to apply other paradigms to enhance automatic and controlled processes. The authors investigated whether activating the stop goal in the go/no-go paradigm is an executively controlled process. More specifically, the authors investigated whether the stop goal can be automatically activated through memory retrieval of consistent associations between the no-go stimulus and stopping. Results show that response inhibition can be achieved through either automatic or controlled processing, depending on the consistency of associations between stimuli and stopping.

Finally to disentangle the contributions of automatic and controlled processes, Debner and Jacoby [39] and Meier, Morger and Graf [40] examined stem-completion test performance in a condition that required subjects not to give as stem-completions any primes they were able to identify and remember [41, 42]. They showed masked primes for a long and for a short time. Priming effect occurs in the short-display condition but not in the long-display condition. The authors interpreted this pattern of results as evidence that the short displays were sufficient to facilitate the subsequent automatic reprocessing of the prime words, but not long enough to permit their consciously controlled processing.

Different paradigms compared here show, as seen above, that they are all useful to better clarify the complex aspects involved in automatic and controlled processes.

## REFERENCES

[1]   Verbruggen, F., & Logan, G.D. (2008). Aftereffects of goal shifting and response inhibition: A comparison of the stop-change and dual-task paradigms. *Quarterly Journal of Experimental Psychology, 61* 1151-1159

[2]   Fisk, A.D., & Schneider, W. (1982). Type of task practice and time-sharing activities predict performance deficits due to alcohol ingestion. Proceedings of the Human Factors Society – 26th Annual meeting, Seattle, WA.

[3]   Shiffrin, R. M., & Schneider, W. (1977). Controlled and automatic human information processing: II: Perceptual learning, automatic attending, and a general theory. *Psychological Review, 84*, 127-190.

[4]   Stroop, J.R. (1935). Studies of interference in serial-verbal reaction. *Journal of Experimental Psychology, 18*, 643-662.

[5]   MacLeod, C.M. (1991). Half a century of research on the Stroop effect: an intregative review. *Psychological Bulletin, 109*, 163-203.

[6]   Jacoby, L. L., Lindsay, D. S., & Hessels, S. (2003). Item-specific control of automatic processes: Stroop process dissociations. *Psychonomic Bulletin & Review, 10*, 634-644.

[7]   Murray, D.J., Mastroddi, J., & Duncan, S. (1972). Selective attention to 'physical" versus "verbal" aspects of coloured words. *Psychonomic Science, 26*, 305-307.

[8]   Hintzman, D.L., Cane, F.A.,Eskridge, V.L., Owens, A.M., Shaft, S.S., & Sparks, M.E. (1972). "Stroop" effect. Input or output phenomenon. *Journal of Experimental Psychology, 95*, 458-459.

[9]   Posner, M.I., & Snyder, C.R.R. (1975). Attention and cognitive control. In R. Solso (ed.), *Information Processing and Cognition: The Loyola Symposium* (pp. 550-585). Hillsdale, N.J.: Lawrence Erlbaum Associates.

[10]  Kiefer, M. (2002). The N400 is modulated by unconsciously perceived masked words: futher wvidence for a spreading activaction account of N400 priming effects. *Cognitive Brain Research,13*, 27-39.

[11]  Klotz, W. & Neumann, O. (1999). Motor activation without conscious discrimination in metacontrast masking. *Journal of Experimental Psychology: Human Perception & Performance, 25*, 976-992.

[12]  Vorberg D., Mattler U., Heinecke A., Schmidt T., Schwarzbach J. V. (2003). Different time courses for visual perception and action priming. *National Academy of Sciences. Proceedings*, 100, 10, 6275-6280.

[13]  Abrams, R.L., & Greenwald, A.G. (2000). Parts outweigh the whole (word) in uncoscious analysis of meaning. *Psychological Science, 11,* 118-124.

[14]  Damian, M.F. (2001). Congruity effects evoked by subliminally presented primes: automaticity rather than semantic processing. *Journal of Experimental Psychology: Human Perception and Performance, 29,* 154-165.

[15]  Carr, T.K., & Dagenbach, D. (1990). Semantic priming and repetition priming from masked words: evidence for center surround-attention mechanism in percertual recognition. *Journal of Experimental Psychology: learning, memory,and cognition, 16,* 341-350.

[16]  Kiefer, M., & Spitzer, M. (2000). Time course of conscious and unconscious semantic brain activation. *Neuroreport, 11,* 2401-2407.

[17]  Kiefer, M.(2007). Top-down modulation of unconscious "automatic" processes: a gating framework. *Advances in Cognitive Psychology, 3,* 289-306.

[18]  Rolke, B., Heil, M., Streb, J., & Henninghausen, E. (2001). Missed prime words within the attentional blink evoke an N400 semantic priming effects. *Psychophysiology, 38,* 165-174.

[19]  Neely, J. H. (1991). Semantic priming effects in visual word recognition:A selective review of current findings and theories. In D. Besner & G. W. Humphreys (Eds.), *Basic processes in reading:Visual word recognition* (pp. 264–336). Hillsdale, NJ: Erlbaum.

[20]  Merril, E. D. (1992). Attentional resource demands of stimulus encoding for persons with and without mental retardation. *American Journal on Mental Retardation, 97, 1,* 87-98.

[21]  Melnik, L. & Das, J. P. (1992). Measurement of attention deficit: correspondence between rating scale and tests of sustained and selective attention. *American Journal on Mental Retardation, 96, 6,* 599-606.

[22]  Fabio, R.A., & Cossutta, R. (2001). Selezione automatica e modello multimediale in soggetti normali e con ritardo mentale. *Giornale italiano di psicologia, 3,* 557-574.

[23]  Szymura, B., Slabosz, A. & Orzechowski, J., (2001). *Some benefits and costs of the selectivity automatization.* Poster prepared for the 12th Conference of the ESCOP, Edinburgh. 5-8 September 2001.

[24]  Moron, M. (1997). Unpublished MA Thesis. Krakow: Jagiellonian University.

[25]  Fabio, R.A., Losa, S., & Viganò, A. (2003). Processi automatici e controllati nei soggetti con Disturbo da Deficit di Attenzione/Iperattività. Psichiatria dell'Infanzia e dell'Adolescenza, 70, 3, 409-421.

[26]  Brickencamp, R., & Zillmer, E. (1998). The d2 test of attention. (1$^{st}$ US ed.). Seattle, WA: Hogrefe & Publishers.

[27]  Bekker, E.M., Overtoom, C.C., Kooij, J.J., Buitelaar, J.K., Verbaten, M.N. & Kenemans, J.L. (2005). Disentangling deficits in adults with attention-deficit/hyperactivity disorder. Arch Gen Psychiatry, 62, 1129-1136.

[28]  Iaboni, F., Douglas, V.I., & Baker, A.G., (1995). Effects of reward and response costs on inhibition in AHD children. Journal of Abnormal Psychology,104, 232-240.

[29]  McLean, A., Dowson ,J., Toone, B., Young, S., Bazanis, E. & Robbins, T.W. (2004): Characteristic neurocognitive profile associated with adult attentiondeficit/ hyperactivity disorder. Psychol Med, 34, 681– 692.

[30]  Schachar, R. & Logan, G. D. (1990) Impulsivity and inhibitory control in normal development and childhood psychopathology. Developmental Psychology, 25, 710-720.

[31]  Kramer, A.F., Humphry, D.G., Larish, J.F., Logan, G.D., & Strayler, D.L. (1994). Aging and inibition: Beyond a unitary view of inhibitory processing in attention. Psychology and Aging, 9, 491-512.

[32]  Levin, H.S., Culhane, K.A., Hartmann, J., Evankovich, K., Mattson, A.J., Harward, H., Ringholz, G., Ewing-Cobbs, L., & Fletcher, J.M. (1991). Developmental changes in performance on tests of purported frontal lobe functioning. Developmental Neuropsychology, 7, 377-395.

[33]  Nielson, K.A., Langenecker, S.A., & Garavan, H. (2002) .Differences in the functional neuroanatomy of inhibitory control across the adult lifespan. Psychology & Aging, 17(issue1), 56-71.

[34]  Williams, B.R., Ponesse, J.S., Schachar, R.J., Logan, G.D., & Tannock, R. (1999). Development of inhibitory control across the life span. Developmental Psychology, 35, 205-213.

[35]  Logan, G.D., Schachar, R.J., & Tannock, R. (1997).impulsivity and inhibitory control. Psychological Science, 8, 60-64.

[36]  Reynolds, B., Ortengren, A., Richards J.B., & De Wit, H. (2006). Dimensions of impulsive behavior: Personality and behavioral measures. Pers Indiv Differ, 40, 305-315.

[37]  Logan, G.D. (1981). Attention,automaticity and the ability to stop a speeded choice response. In J. Long, & A.Baddeley (Eds.), Attention and performance IX (pp.205-222). Hillsdale, N. J.: Erlbaum.

[38] Logan, G.D., & Cowan, W.B. (1984). On the ability to inhibit thought and action: A theory of an act of control. *Psychological Review, 91*, 295-327.

[39] Debner, J. A., & Jacoby, L. L. (1994). Unconscious perception: Attention, awareness, and control. *Journal of Experimental Psychology: Learning, Memory and Cognition, 20*, 304–317.

[40] Meier, B., Morger, V., & Graff, P. (2003). Competition between automatic and controlled processes. *Consciousness and Cognition, 12*, 309-319.

[41] Jacoby, L. L. (1991). A process dissociation framework: Separating automatic from intentional uses of memory. *Journal of Memory and Language, 30*, 513–541.

[42] Jacoby, L. L., & Whitehouse, K. (1989). An illusion of memory: False recognition influenced by unconscious perception. *Journal of Experimental Psychology: General, 118*, 126–135.

[43] Merikle, P. M., Joordens, S., & Stolz, J. A. (1995). Measuring the relative magnitude of unconscious influences. *Consciousness and Cognition, 4*, 422–439.

[44] Hasher, L., & Zacks, R. (1979). Automatic and effortful processes in memory. *Journal of Experimental Psychology: General, 108*, 356-388.

[45] Lavie, N. (1995). Perceptual load as a necessary condition for selective attention. *J. Exp. Psychol. Hum. Percept. Perform. 21*, 451-468.

# Chapter 3

# NEUROLOGICAL BASES OF AUTOMATIC AND CONTROLLED PROCESSES

## ABSTRACT

Recent years have witnessed a mounting interest in the impact of the neurological basis of most cognitive processes. Methods such as positron emission tomography (PET) and functional magnetic resonance imaging (fMRI) allow the volumetric variations in regional cerebral blood flow that are related with cognitive activity to be indexed with millimeter-level spatial resolution. Much of the interest on cognitive processes has focused on two phenomena: stimulus-driven or bottom-up effects on attentional selection, and goal-driven or top-down influences. This chapter examines the current status of research on the neurological bases of automatic and controlled processes with reference to fMRI methodologies, to EEG and ERP studies, aiming at clarifying what is known about each of these phenomena and why they are both worth knowing about.

## LOCI OF AUTOMATIC AND CONTROLLED PROCESSES – NEUROIMAGING RESEARCH

As seen in the previous chapters, any view on cognition [1, 2, 3] posits the existence of top-down signals that select and coordinate information. These signals are thought to enhance the representations that underlie our conscious perceptions, thoughts, and plans of actions, while inhibiting irrelevant or inappropriate information.

On the other hand, many brain processes can work without top-down control: well-learned, habitual behaviors can be executed automatically, and unexpected events can automatically grab our attention and enter our awareness. Top-down control is necessary, however, when we need to ignore distractions or to inhibit reflexive, prepotent responses and when habitual behaviors cannot be used, as in novel or difficult situations.

Perhaps the best understood example of top-down control is selective visual attention, that is, the ability to voluntarily focus our awareness on relevant stimuli and ignore irrelevant stimuli. This ability is critical because our capacity for visual processing is severely limited; at any given moment, we can only fully process a small portion of a scene. Intelligent behaviour thus depends on suppressing reflexive orientation to physically salient inputs and on selectively gathering inputs that are behaviourally relevant. Various accounts of selective attention have held that it can be focused on relevant visual field locations and objects, and that processing of relevant visual attributes is enhanced, whereas processing of irrelevant attributes is suppressed.

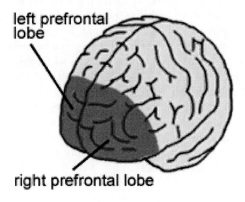

Figure 1. Frontal lobes

Selective attention has long been thought to be an important prefrontal function. Damage to the prefrontal (PF) cortex in humans can cause deficits in sustained attention and detection of novel events [4, 5; 6]. Further, deficits on complex tasks after PF damage have been thought to reflect a dysfunction in switching attention between different visual features of a task, between different sets of abstract behavior-guiding rules, or both [7]. Similarly, PF lesions in monkeys can result in deficits in shifting attention between different stimulus dimensions [8].

Desimone and Duncan [9] have proposed a biologically plausible model to explain these phenomena. According to biased competition, neurons in the extrastriate visual cortex that represent different visual field locations and objects are mutually inhibitory. Top-down signals are excitatory and represent the item to be attended. These bias signals increase activity of neurons that process the relevant information and, by virtue of the mutual inhibition, suppress activity of neurons processing irrelevant information. Top-down signals are thought to derive from maintained activity of the task-relevant information, activity that conveys information about the sought-after item.

In this chapter, neurophysiological studies relevant to topdown attentional selection (controlled) by biased competition will be discussed, focusing on the properties of neurons in the prefrontal cortex, a brain region thought to be involved in top-down control and to provide the bias signals that mediate attentional selection. Reflexive systems will be also discussed.

Satpute and Lieberman [10] point out that reflexive systems correspond to automatic processes and include the amygdala, basal ganglia, ventromedial prefrontal cortex, dorsal anterior cingulate cortex, and lateral temporal cortex. Reflective systems correspond to controlled processes and include lateral prefrontal cortex, posterior parietal cortex, medial prefrontal cortex, rostral anterior cingulate cortex, and the hippocampus and surrounding medial temporal lobe region.

Luu, Tucker and Stripling [11] also outlined that neuro imaging studies have suggested there may be direct neural correlates of the reduced demands for controlled processes, as evidenced by decreased demands on brain activity resulting from increasing practice with task performance.

Given that frontal lobe activity is thought to be particularly important to goal representations and providing control- related outputs [12], it is theoretically important that both meta-analysis of fMRI studies and new experiments have suggested a specific decrease in frontal lobe activity (bilateral dorsal frontal, left ventral prefrontal, anterior cingulate cortex, left insular regions) as participants become more practiced in task performance [13] .

Functional neuroimaging studies of hemodynamic responses during arbitrary visuomotor association learning have identified the involvement of the anterior cingulate sulcus, parahippocampal gyrus, caudate nucleus (i.e., dorsal striatum), inferior frontal gyrus, middle temporal gyrus, dorsal premotor cortex, and parietal cortex [14, 15, 16].These regions appear to overlap substantially with the neural networks implicated in controlled cognitive processes by Chein and Schneider [13], and certain of these structures are closely related to the fast learning corticothalamic-limbic circuit implicated by Gabriel and colleagues in the early stages of discriminant learning.

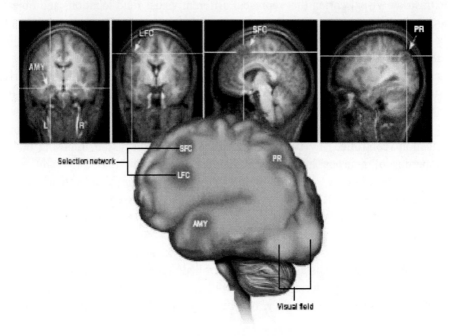

Figure 2. Frontal lobe activity when controlled processes are actived

Also Schneider and Chein [17] in one study attempt to construct a model of automatic and controlled processes and consider three basic predictions that can be tested through functional neuroimaging research.

The first regards the Control System. As described above, the Control System plays a central role during early CM task learning, but a considerably reduced role late in CM learning. Accordingly, a first prediction is that the neural substrates of the Control System should be identifiable in a contrast of brain activity produced during performance of a consistent task early in practice to that produced later in practice.

More generally, areas implementing Control System processes are expected to be active when tasks require effortful and intentional processing, and to decrease activity as automaticity develops.

A second prediction stems from the fact that the Control System provides executive resources for all tasks before they are automatized. Consequently, the second prediction is that brain regions supporting controlled processing should be active in novice performance across a wide range of tasks and materials.

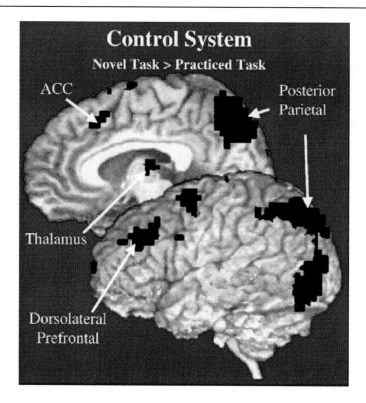

Figure 3. FMRI image of brain regions in which activity decreases with practise of CM [17]. The black areas indicate the reduction of activity after practise

The third prediction they consider is that, since automatic processing is based on the operation of the same modules that were involved during earlier controlled processing of the same task, the brain regions that remain active following extensive consistent practice should also have been active during early practice on the task.

## IS THE PREFRONTAL CORTEX THE ONLY LOCUS FOR TOP-DOWN SIGNAL AND CONTROLLED PROCESSES?

As Miller, Erickson & Desimone [18] point out the prefrontal (PF) cortex is associated with a wide range of "executive" functions critical for complex behavior, such as problem solving, planning, selecting action, and working memory. Consistent with an "executive" role in brain function are the extensive interconnections between the PF cortex and many other brain regions [19, 20, 21, 22, 23]. It should be noted, however, that the prefrontal cortex is unlikely either to be the only region involved in top-down control or to act alone. For example, some studies implicate frontostriatal loops in topdown control of attention [24].

According to the biased competition model, the role of the prefrontal cortex in visual attention is to provide activity that biases competition in the visual cortex in favor of neurons representing that information. The PF cortex is thought to provide "attentional templates" by maintaining activity that conveys information about the sought-after item. This ability is typically studied in delay tasks in which a single stimulus is presented as a cue and then, after a delay, monkeys make a response based on that cue. During the delay, many PF neurons show high levels of often cue-specific activity [18, 25, 26]. Human imaging studies also indicate high levels of sustained PF activity during such tasks [27, 28].

This "delay activity" can convey information about stimulus identity and location, and thus might play a role in directing attention to relevant form or color attributes, and or to particular locations. Other properties of prefrontal neurons also seem ideal for a role in voluntarily directing attention. They can select and integrate information from diverse sources and can maintain activity about this information in the face of distractions. Further, the PF cortex seems to play a central role in the "executive" brain functions that determine what is relevant and needs attending. This may be mediated by PF mechanisms that acquire and represent behaviour guiding rules and behavioral context. The dorsolateral prefrontal cortex (DLPFC) is frequently cited as the locus of executive processes [29]. Furthermore, axons from many different cortical regions project ultimately to the PFC (via the intralaminar nuclei of the thalamus), particularly the dorsolateral portion, thereby providing the necessary pathway through which output signals transmitted from all over the brain can converge on this centralized processor [30]. The DLPFC is also implicated in guiding the sequential execution of operations during controlled processing [31], as would be expected of a region behaving as the Goal Processor. The GP should be active when a novel task is encountered (because a novel task requires that a new sequencing procedure be developed), and for tasks that require variable binding (e.g., VM search). Tasks that have a high workload or require the planning and ordering of many sequential operations should also engage this brain region. Broadly, the prefrontal cortex again fits this profile. The prefrontal cortex has been shown to be active in a wide variety of cognitive tasks [32], and Shallice and Burgess [33] have argued that planning is one of the primary functions of this brain region. Increases in activation with workload are also often reported in the prefrontal cortex [27, 34], and complex cognitive tasks [35, 36] often elicit extensive PFC activity.

# ERP's Studies

The study of automaticity in information-processing is facilitated by the recording of ERPs, as they provide a means of determining the extent to which to-be-ignored stimuli are processed.

Although some studies have emphasized the importance of the ACC (anterior cingulated cortex) in action monitoring [37], many of the human findings of error-related negativities (response-locked ERNs) or medial frontal negativities (stimulus-locked MFN or N2) have shown strong responses in medial frontal cortex when the subject's expectancies are violated.

These results may be consistent with more elementary learning processes; discrepancy or conflict detection is a requirement for behavioural adjustments. Indeed, it is through the detection of discrepancies between what is expected, given a particular action, and what actually happened that new learning occurs [38]. According to an influential theory of medial frontal control of cognitive conflict, the ERN (error related negativity) reflects the activity of a learning system that relies on prediction errors (Holroyd and Coles, 2002).

In a recent work Luu, Tuckera and Stripling [37] presented participants with an associative ("code learning") task, in which they needed to discover an arbitrary mapping of stimuli (digits or spatial location) with key presses of the correct hand and finger, or with no response. The authors hypothesized that the learning process would engage frontal lobe activity implicated in controlled cognitive processes (anterior ventral network). In contrast, as participants learned this task, the consolidation of a cognitive context for performance would be indexed by an increasingly robust P300 or Late Positive Complex (LPC), generated in medial temporal, posterior cingulate, and parietal cortices, thus reflecting the more automatic process typical of expert performance.

Results of their study are very important and give information to progressive engagement of brain networks in the process of learning. In early learning stages, when participants are still trying to associate visual information with appropriate responses, lateralized negativities originated with the onset of the N1. These lateralized negativities (left for digit code, right for spatial code) spread from lateral temporal recording sites to inferior anterior sites, peaking at approximately 390 ms post-target. The authors measured the peak of this effect as the LIAN (lateral inferior anterior negativity). After participants learned the task, there were three prominent changes identified in the ERPs. The first was a reduction in LIAN amplitude, particularly for spatial targets.

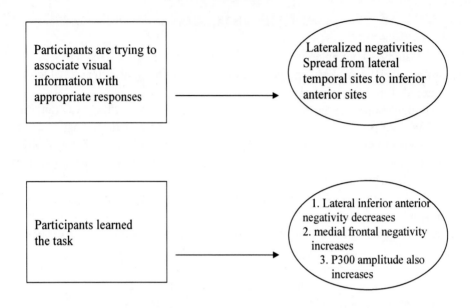

Figure 4. The Luu, Tuckera and Stripling 's paradigm

This confirms the hypothesis of a decrease in frontal contributions to controlled processes as learning progresses. The other two changes involved increases in MFN the medial frontal negativity and P300 amplitude in the post-learned state. Whereas the increase in P300 was predicted and is consistent with previous research, the increase in the MFN with learning was unexpected. Results reveal that the transition between not knowing what to do and performing appropriate actions in context (learning) is marked by differential decreases in right frontal lobe activation and increased activation in the ACC and posterior networks of the temporal lobe, PCC, and parietal cortex.

Unlike fMRI studies, EEG and ERP methodologies show the time course of brain activity.

The results revealed substantial temporal overlap between processes indexed by three ERP components. The LIAN is initiated quite early and appears to be a continuation of the neural activity that extends along the extent of the temporal lobe, perhaps reflecting memory operations in occipitotemporal networks. The strong activation of inferior frontal and anterior temporal regions (at the peak of the LIAN) overlaps temporally with ACC (MFN), PCC, medial temporal, and parietal activations. The data also suggest that the course of learning related to the processes regulated by these structures is quite different. Activity recorded from frontal and temporal structures, at least the right-hemisphere response associated with spatial targets, decrease at a faster rate than activity in the ACC. It remains to be seen whether left-hemisphere activity (indexed by the LIAN) and ACC activity associated with conflict monitoring would decrease, as expected, with extended practice.

These electrophysiological signs of early learning processes are followed by a gradual development of the P300, reflecting activation within medial and posterior networks of the temporal lobe, as well as associated networks of the posterior cingulate and parietal cortices. The involvement of these posterior cortical structures marks the transition to the later stage of learning and perhaps the onset of automaticity.

In another work, Muller-Gass, Macdonald, Schröger, Sculthorpe and Campbell [39] hypothesised that the P3a, an ERP component is believed to index the occurrence of an attentional capture [40]. Within the context of distraction, the P3a is elicited by task-irrelevant stimuli or stimulus information occurring in an easily distinguished channel compared to task-relevant stimuli. The processing of the distractor may come at a cost for task performance because attention is switched from the task-relevant to the irrelevant channel. This is particularly the case when the temporal proximity between the occurrence of distractor and the task-relevant information is   short [41]. The P3a follows a deviant stimulus that also elicits an earlier additional negativity, composed of an enhanced N1 and/or a mismatch negativity (MMN) component.

N1 is enhanced when the deviant stimulus represents a frequency or locus change, or an intensity or duration (for brief stimuli) increment; whereas MMN is elicited by a violation in the predictability of a stimulus sequence [42]. The strength (amplitude) of the N1 and MMN signals is a determining factor in the generation and size of the P3a [43, 44]. The N1 and MMN reflect automatic processes, in as much as these components are still generated when attention is effectively withdrawn from the eliciting stimuli [42, 45]. The processes underlying N1 and MMN thus do not require attention for their occurrence; however, they may be attenuated or enhanced based on the availability of attentional capacity (N1 effect, [46, 47]see Hillyard et al., 1973; for a recent reviewon MMN and attention, see *Muller-Gass=et al., 2006*). They can thus be conceived, at least under some circumstances, as weakly automatic processes. Hackley [48] suggests that the transition from strong to weak automaticity in auditory information processing may occur as early as 15 ms. There are however ERP components (e.g. PN, N2b) prior to the time of P3a that are attention-dependent and reflect controlled processing.

## AUDITORY STIMULI AND AUTOMATIC
## AND CONTROLLED PROCESSES

A study of Muller-Gass et al. [39] examines whether the processes underlying the auditory P3a are of automatic or controlled nature.

The primary aim of the study of Muller-Gass et al. [39] was to examine whether the P3a was automatically generated; that is, whether the processes underlying the generation of the P3a operate without attention (i.e. an automatic process), or whether these processes can potentially be abolished by the withdrawal of attention (i.e. a controlled process). In order to test this, they employed a task that requires highly-focused attention, thereby ensuring that the P3a-eliciting stimuli consistently occur outside of the focus of attention.

In their study Muller-Gass et al. [39] optimised the experimental conditions in order to maximise the need and capability to highly focus attention on the visual task. The need was established by using a difficult continuous tracking task, which promotes the selective processing of task-relevant visual information. This task required subjects to track and respond to target objects and ignore identical non-target objects, as they moved randomly around a rectangular space [49]. Furthermore, in order to allow the subject to more readily ignore the auditory sequence, they employed a very rapid (on average every 244 ms) and random auditory presentation rate. In the study the likelihood of obtaining a P3a was also maximised by using deviant stimuli (a small intensity increment and a large intensity decrement) that are known to elicit a large P3a [47, 50]. If the P3a is elicited under these stringent conditions, then the processes underlying the P3a are automatic, not reliant on centralised capacity, as this capacity is consumed by the demands of the difficult continuous visual task [51].

More specifically, Muller-Gass et al. [39] investigated whether the auditory P3a is an attention-independent component, that is, whether it can still be elicited under highly-focused selective attention to a different (visual) channel and whether the auditory P3a can be modulated by the demands of the visual diversion task. Subjects performed a continuous visual tracking task that varied in difficulty, based on the number of objects to-be-tracked. Task-irrelevant auditory stimuli were presented at very rapid and random rates concurrently to the visual task. The auditory sequence included rare increments ($+10$ dB) and decrements ($-20$ dB) in intensity relative to the frequently-presented standard stimulus.

Results show that the auditory deviant stimuli elicited a significant P3a during the most difficult visual task, when conditions were optimised to prevent attentional slippage to the auditory channel. This finding suggests that the elicitation of the auditory P3a does not require available central capacity, and confirms the automatic nature of the processes underlying this ERP component. Moreover, the difficulty of the visual task did not modulate either themismatch negativity (MMN) or the P3a but did have an effect on a late (350–400ms) negativity, an ERP deflection perhaps related to a subsequent evaluation of the auditory change. Together, these results imply that the auditory P3a could reflect a strongly-automatic process, one that does not require and is not modulated by attention.

## CONCLUSION

In this chapter the current status of research on the neurological bases of automatic and controlled processes with reference to fMRI methodologies and ERP studies was presented.

Both approaches seem to converge in outlining two qualitatively different activations underlying automatic and controlled processes.

From fMRI it follows that reflexive systems correspond to automatic processes and include the amygdala, basal ganglia, ventromedial prefrontal cortex, dorsal anterior cingulate cortex, and lateral temporal cortex. Reflective systems correspond to controlled processes and include lateral prefrontal cortex, posterior parietal cortex, medial prefrontal cortex, rostral anterior cingulate cortex, and the hippocampus and surrounding medial temporal lobe region.

Selective attention has long been thought to be an important prefrontal function. Damage to the prefrontal (PF) cortex in humans can cause deficits in sustained attention and detection of novel events. Further, deficits on complex tasks after PF damage have been thought to reflect a dysfunction in switching attention between different visual features of a task, between different sets of abstract behavior-guiding rules, or both. Luu, Tucker and Stripling [37] also outlined that neuro imaging studies have suggested there may be direct neural correlates of the reduced demands for controlled processes, as evidenced by decreased demands on brain activity resulting from increasing practice with task performance, and that frontal lobe activity is thought to be particularly important to goal representations and providing control- related outputs [12]. It is theoretically important that meta-analysis of fMRI studies and new experiments have suggested a specific decrease in frontal lobe activity (bilateral dorsal frontal, left ventral prefrontal, anterior cingulate cortex, left insular regions) as participants become more practiced in task performance.

A question was proposed in this chapter and was whether prefrontal cortex is the only locus for top-down signal and controlled processes. Different authors conclude that the dorsolateral prefrontal cortex (DLPFC) is frequently cited as the locus of executive processes [29]. Furthermore, axons from many different cortical regions project ultimately to the PFC (via the intralaminar nuclei of the thalamus), particularly the dorsolateral portion, thereby providing the necessary pathway through which output signals transmitted from all over the brain can converge on this centralized processor [17].

With reference to ERP studies, a study of Muller-Gass et al. [39] examines whether the processes underlying the auditory P3a are of automatic or controlled nature. Results show that these electrophysiological signs of early learning processes are followed by a gradual development of the P300, reflecting activation within medial and posterior networks of the temporal lobe, as well as associated networks of the posterior cingulate and parietal cortices. The involvement of these posterior cortical structures marks the transition to the later stage of learning and perhaps the onset of automaticity. Also with reference to auditory stimuli, findings suggest that the elicitation of the auditory P3a does not require available central capacity, and confirms the automatic nature of the processes underlying this ERP component.

# REFERENCES

[1] Baddeley, A.D. (1986). *Working memory.* Oxford: Oxford University Press.
[2] Norman, D.E., & Shallice, T. (1986). Attention to action: Willed and automatic control of behaviour. In R. Davison, G. Schwartz, & D. Shapiro (Eds.), *Consciousness and self-regulation:Advances in research and theory.* New York: Plenum.
[3] Johnson, M.K., & Hirst, W. (1991). Processing subsystems of memory. In R.G. Lister, & H.J. Weingartner (Eds.), *Perspectives in cognitive neuroscience.* (pp. 197-217). New York: Oxford University Press.
[4] Knight, R. T. (1984). Decreased response to novel stimuli after prefrontal lesions in man. *Electroencephalogr. Clin. Neurophysiol. ,59,* 9–20.
[5] Knight, R. T. (1991). Evoked potential studies of attention capacity in human frontal lobe lesions. In H. S. Levin, H. M. Eisenberg, & A. L. Benton (Eds.), *Frontal lobe function and dysfunction* (pp. 139-153). New York: Oxford University Press.

[6]   Stuss, D.T., & Benson, D.F. (1986). *The frontal lobes*. New York: Raven Press.
[7]   Owen, A.M., Roberts, A.C., Polkey, C.E., Sahakian, B.J., & Robbins T.W. *(*1991*)* Extra-dimensional versus intra-dimensional set-shifting performance following frontal lobe excisions, temporal lobe excisions or amygdalohippocampectomy in man. *Neuropsychologia, 29,* 993–1006.
[8]   Dias, R., Robbins, T.W., & Roberts, A.C., (1996). Dissociation in prefrontal cortex of affective and attentional shifts. *Nature, 380,* 69-72.
[9]   Desimone, R., & Duncan, J. (1995). Neural mechanisms of selective visual attention. *Annu Rev Neurosci, 18,* 193-222.
[10]  Satpute, A.B., & Lieberman, M. D. (2006). Integrating automatic and controlled processing into neurocognitive models of social cognition. *Brain Research,* 1079, 86-97.
[11]  Luu, P., Tucker, D. M.,& Stripling, R. (2007). Neural mechanisms for learning actions in context. *Brainresearch, 1179,* 89 – 105.
[12]  Miller, E.K., & Cohen, J.D. (2001). An integrative theory of prefrontal cortex function. *Annu. Rev. Neurosci, 24,* 167–202.
[13]  Chein, J.M.,& Schneider, W. (2005). Neuroimaging studies of practice-related change: fMRI and meta-analytic evidence of a domain general control network for learning. Cogn. *Brain Res,* 25, 607–623.
[14]  Toni, I., & Passingham, R.E. (1999). Prefrontal-basal ganglia pathways are involved in the learning of arbitrary visuomotor associations: a pet study. *Exp. Brain Res, 127,* 19–32.
[15]  Toni, I., Ramnani, N., Josephs, O., Ashburner, J., & Passingham, R.E. (2001). Learning arbitrary visuomotor associations: temporal dynamic of brain activity. *NeuroImage,14,* 1048–1057.
[16]  Wise, S.P., & Murray, E.A. (2000) Arbitrary associations between antecedents and actions. *Trends Neurosci 23,* 271–276.
[17]  Schneider, W., & Chein, J.M. (2003). Controlled and automatic processes: behaviour, theory and biological mecanisms. *Cognitive Science,* 27, 525-559.
[18]  Miller, E.K., Erickson, C.A., & Desimone, R. (1996). Neural mechanism of visual working memory in prefrontal cortex of the macaque. *J Neurosci, 16,* 154-5167.
[19]  Pandya, D.N., & Yeterian, E. (1990). Prefrontal cortex in relation to other cortical areas in Rhesus monkey: Architecture and connections. *Progress in Brain Research, 85,* 63-94.

[20] Pandya, D. N., & Barnes, C.L. (1987).Architecture and connections of the frontal lobe. In E. Perecman (Ed), *The Frontal Lobes Revisited* ( pp 41-72). New York : The IRNN Press.

[21] Cavada, C., & Goldman-Rakic, P.S. (1989). Posterior parietal cortex in rhesus monkey: Evidence for segregated cortical networks linking sensory and limbic areas with the frontal lobe. *J. Comp. Neurol., 287,* 422-445.

[22] Preuss, T. M., & Goldman-Rakic, P.S. (1989). Connections of the ventral granular frontal cortex of macaques with perisylvian premotor and somatosensory areas: Anatomical evidence for somatic representation in primate frontal association cortex. *J. Comp. Neurol.* 282, 293-316.

[23] Webster, M.J., Bachevalier, J.,& Ungerleider, L.G. (1994) Connections of inferior temporal areas TEO and TE with parietal and frontal cortex in macaque monkeys. *Cereb. Cortex ,4,* 470-483.

[24] Robbins, T.W., & Rogers, R.D. (2000). Functioning of frontostrial anatomical "loops" in mechanism of cognitive control. *Attention and Performance XVIII : control of cognitive processess* (pp. 475-509). Cambridge MA: MIT Press.

[25] Rainer, G., Asaad, W. E., & Miller, E.K. (1998a). Memory fields of neurons in the primate prefrontal cortex. *Proceedings of the national academy of sciences U.S.A., 95,* 15008- 15013.

[26] Rainer, G., Asaad, W. E., & Miller, E.K. (1998b). Selective representation of relevant information by neurons in the primate prefrontal cortex. *Nature, 393,* 577-579

[27] Cohen, L.G., Celnik, P., Pascual-Leone, A., Corwell, B., & Falz, L. (1997). Functional relevance of cross-modal plasticity in blind humans. *Nature, 389,*180–183.

[28] Courtney, S.M., Ungerleider, L.G., Keil, K.,& Haxby, J.V. (1997). Transient and sustained activity in a distributed neural system for human working memory. *Nature, 386,* 608-611.

[29] Robert, T.W., Robbins, Y.L.,& Weiskrantz, L. (1998). *The prefrontal cortex executive and cognitive functions* (Eds.). New York: Oxford University Press.

[30] Schneider, W. (1999). Working memory in a multilevel hybrid connectionist control architecture (CAP2). In A. Miyake & P. Shah (Eds.), *Models of working memory: Mechanisms of active maintenance and executive control* (pp. 340–374). New York, NY: Cambridge University Press.

[31]  Schneider, W., & Oliver, W. L. (1991). An instructable connectionist/control architecture: Using rule-based instructions to accomplish connectionist learning in a human time scale. In K. Van Lehn (Ed.), *Architectures for intelligence: The 22nd Carnegie Mellon symposium on cognition* (pp. 113–145). Hillsdale, NJ: Lawrence Erlbaum.

[32]  Cabeza, R.,& Nyberg, L. (2000). Imaging cognition II: An empirical review of 275 pet and fMRI. *Studies. J. Cogn Neurosci,12,* 1-47.

[33]  Shallice, T.,& Burgess, P.W. (1996). The domain of supervisory processes and temporal organization of behaviour. *Philosophical Transictions of the royal society of London B, 351,* 1405-1412.

[34]  D'Esposito, M., Detre, J. A., Alsop, D. C., & Shin, R. K. (1995). The neural basis of the central executive system of working memory. *Nature, 1378,* 279–281.

[35]  Prabhakaran,V., Smith, J.A.L., Desmond, J.E., Glover, G.H., & Gabrieli, J.D.E. (1997b). Neural Substrates of Fluid Reasoning: An fMRI Study of Neocortical Activation during Performance of the Raven's Progressive Matrices Test. *Cognitive Psychology,* 33, 43-63.

[36]  Fincham, J.M., Carter, C.S.,Van,V.V., Stenger, V.A., & Anderson, J.R. (2002). Neural mechanism of planning: a computational analysis using event-related fMRI. *Proc Natl Acad Sci USA,99,* 3346-3351.

[37]  Luu, P., & Tucker, D.M. (2003). Self-regulation and the executive functions: electrophysiological clues. In A. Zani, & A.M. Preverbio (Eds.), *The Cognitive Electrophysiology of Mind and Brain.*(pp. 199–223). San Diego: Academic Press.

[38]  Rescorla, R.A., & Wagner, A.R. (1972). A theory of pavlovian conditioning: variations in the effectiveness of reinforcement and nonreinforcement. In A.H. Black, & W.F. Prokasy (Eds.), *Classical Conditioning II: Current Research and Theory.* (pp. 64–99). New York : Appleton-Century-Corfts.

[39]  Muller-Gass, A., Macdonald, M., Schröger, E., Sculthorpe, L.,& Campbell, K.B. (2007). Evidence for the auditory P3a reflecting an authomatic process: elicitation during highly-focused continuous visual attention. *Brain Research,1170,* 71-78.

[40]  Escera, C., Alho,K., Schroger, E.,& Winkler, I. (2000). Involuntary attention and distractibility as evaluated with event-related brain potentials. *Audiol. Neurootol.,5,*151-166.

[41]  Schroger, E. (1996). A neural mechanism for involuntary attention shifts to changes in auditory stimulation. *Journal of Cognitive Neuroscience, 8,* 527-539.

[42]  Näätänen, R.Y.,Picton,T. (1987). The N1 wave of the human electric and magnetic response to sound: a review and a analysis of the component structure. *Psychophysiology,24*, 375-425.

[43]  Berti, S., Roeber, U., & Schro"ger, E. (2004). Bottom-up influences on working memory: behavioral and electrophysiological distraction varies with distractor strength. *Exp Psychol, 51*, 249–57.

[44]  Yago, E., Escera, C., Alho, K., & Giard, M.H. (2001). Cerebral mechanisms underlying orienting of attention towards auditory frequency changes. *Neuroreport, 12, 11*, 2583-2587.

[45]  Woldorff, M.G., Fox, P.T., Matzke, M., Lancaster,J.L., Veevaswamy,S., Zamaripa, F., Seabolt, M., Glass, T., Gao, J.H., Martin, C.C., & Jerabek, P. (1997) . Retinotopic organization of early visual spatial attention effects as revealed by PET and ERPS. *Hum. Brain. Map., 5*, 280-286.

[46]  Hillyard, S.A., Hink, R.F., Schwent, V.L., Picton, T.W., (1973). Electrical signs of selective attention in the human brain. *Science, 182*, 177-179.

[47]  Muller-Gass, A., Stelmarck, R.,& Campbell, K. B. (2006). The effect of visual task difficulty and attentional direction on the detection of acoustic change as indexed by the mismatch negativity. *Brain Res, 1078*, 112-130.

[48]  Hackley, S. (1993). An evaluation of the automaticity of sensory processing using event-related potentials and brain-stem reflexes. *Psychophysiology, 30*, 415-428.

[49]  Pylyshyn,Z. W.,& Storm, R.W. (1998). Tracking multiple independent targets: evidence for a parallel tracking mechanism. *Spatial Vision, 3*, 179-197.

[50]  Rinne, T., Sarkka, A., Degerman, A., Schroger, E., & Alho, K. (2006). Two separate mechanisms underlie auditory change detection and involuntary control of attention. *Brain Res, 1077*,135-143.

[51]  Arnell, K.M.,& Jolicoeur, P. (1999). The attentional blink across stimulus modalities: evidence for central processing limitations. *Journal of experimental psychology:human perception and performance,25*, 1-19.

*Chapter 4*

# UTILITY AND LIMIT OF AUTOMATIZATION

## ABSTRACT

Automatization may present both negative and positive aspects. The aim of this chapter is to analyse whether automatization is simply elegant and economical or it may also adds costs and limits in human performance. To begin, the advantages to having two different processing modes is considered, in effect dual processing mechanisms would likely not have evolved unless there were survival advantages to having both modes of processing. Secondly, benefits of automatization are considered: the greatest advantage of automatic over controlled processes is that they operate more rapidly and can occur in parallel, they are also fast, effortless, autonomous and error-free. Moreover costs of automaticity are analysed, they inhere in the lack of flexibility and control that results when we learn too well and are not conscious of doing some tasks. In the concluding section some thoughts are offered about the fact that there is no clear distinction but a gradation between the two processes and their implication about costs and benefits.

## ADVANTAGES AND DISADVANTAGES OF AUTOMATIC OVER CONTROLLED PROCESSES

As seen above in the first three chapters, automatization refers to acquiring the ability to run without monitoring. As Saling and Phillips [1] point out automatic processes, rather than merely being faster than controlled processes, are instead economical and elegant, occurring without uncertainty or hesitation and although automaticity is seemingly faster at a behavioural level, in the form of more efficient behaviour, this cannot be equated with faster processing at a neural level. As seen in the third chapter with the acquisition of automaticity there is a decrease in global activation or a shift in activation, particularly from cortical regions to subcortical areas. Thus automatic processing is performed differently from controlled processing, apparently employing different, superior algorithms, which in some cases are explicit and in other cases are yet to be documented. In this chapter the aim is to analyse advantages and disadvantages of automatic over controlled processes.

Before considering benefits and limits of automatic and controlled processes, it is important to underline the advantages to having two different processing modes [2].

Dual processing mechanisms would likely not have evolved unless there were survival advantages to having both modes of processing. Schneider and Chein [2] assume that automatic and controlled processing are two qualitatively different forms of processing that provide complementary benefits. In their model, in which the authors show a simulation of automatic and controlled processes, they suggest that a single process alone cannot provide both the fast learning of controlled processing and the high speed parallel robust processing of automatic processing. So, although it may be less parsimonious to assume two different modes of processing, we argue that there are sufficient survival advantages to a two-process system over a unitary architecture to have allowed a dual-process system to evolve.

From the authors' point of view the survival advantages to having both controlled and automatic processing are analogous to the non-overlapping and overlapping benefits of having rod and cone vision. With controlled processing: 1) the fundamentals of new skills can be acquired quickly (e.g., one trial learning to escape when a life threatening stimulus appears), 2) critical stimuli can be attended while ignoring normally relevant stimuli (attend to a child in a crosswalk while inhibiting the prepotent response to accelerate on a green light), 3) variable bindings that allow general operations to be applied to temporarily relevant stimuli can take place (e.g., after eating a novel food, searching for it in the environment), 4) learning can be passed between individuals by instruction or observation (rather than shaping), and 5) goal directed behavior can be planned and executed.

However, due to the slow execution, high effort, and poor robustness of controlled processing, it can operate on only a small number of stimuli at any time, and any skill acquired during controlled performance may not be sufficiently robust to resist rapid decay or deterioration in the presence of stressors. Further, if a task requires the coordination of many sensory/motor inputs, the slow, resource-limited nature of controlled processing will be a serious limitation (e.g., imagine trying to ski down a difficult slope using verbal rules to plan and execute motor movements). Despite taking a long time to acquire, automatic processing has the advantages of being robust under stress.

## BENEFITS

Schneider and Shiffrin point out that the greatest advantage of automatic over controlled processes is that they operate more rapidly and can occur in parallel. Automatic processing is also fast [3, 4], effortless [5, 6, 4, ] , autonomous [5, 6, 7] and error-free. It can be accomplished simultaneously with other cognitive processes without interference, it is not limited by attention capacity and it can be unconscious or involuntary.

Consequently automatic processes do not need constant guidance or monitoring, and therefore use minimal attention capacity. The fact that many of our behaviours become automatic is beneficial. If all our actions required conscious thought, we would spend time planning every step instead of just "walking". Everything would take as much time and be as difficult to do as the first time we did it [8].

In other words, automaticity allows a familiar and comfortable interaction with our environment. With experience we develop habits:; when we go to university for example, we know automatically how things are supposed to go. We go in, we say hallo to the security man, we have lessons, we write down notes and then we can go home. It is like going there for the first time and thinking "what happened the last time I came here? Why are people writing notes?". We automatically know the proper assumption? of the situation based on our experience. As Weatley and Wegner [8] underline, this automatic activation of norms makes the world a much more predictable place.

Another field in which we can see positive effects of automatization is the learning of new skills. For example a study of Parasuraman, Hilburn, Molloy and Singh [9] examined the effects of short-cycle adaptive automation and practice on performance-of flight-related functions in a multi-task environment. Twenty four non pilot subjects were tested on a PC-based flight- simulation task that included three primary flight functions - tracking, monitoring, and fuel management. Each function could be automated or performed manually. The results provide preliminary evidence that dynamic automation shifts over short cycles, of the type likely in adaptive systems, performance benefits with no evidence of costs to performance following the return to manual control. Benefits are realized despite the added workload of supervisory control of automated functions. However, training procedures other than simple practice may be necessary to maximize and maintain the performance benefits associated with adaptive automation. These results suggest that adaptive automation, or adaptive function allocation maximize the benefits associated with cockpit automation while maintaining pilot involvement, enhancing situation awareness, and regulating workload.

# COSTS

On the other hand, there are several claims about the role of automatization. A first claim comes from Phillips and Triggs [10] and is relevant from a methodological point of view. The authors underline that the concept of automaticity arose in the context of explaining observations that could not be accounted for by prevailing models of attention such as information theorem, bottleneck models of attention and capacity theory. Thus, the invocation of automaticity is post hoc. Furthermore, since automaticity is defined in terms of the behaviour to be explained, it is plagued by circularity. Automaticity is used to refer to a family of processes which share only the lack of some or a subset of these features. Automaticity, then, is a negatively defined concept: an absence of at least one key quality of conscious control.

From a more substantial point of view one of the disadvantages of automatic over controlled processes is that the ability may become stereotypic, we can for example give characterizations of persons based on their membership of a particular group (e.g., Asian, Jewish, Southern, etc.) [11] and unavailable to conscious awareness [12] . For example one such pitfall comes from thinking about things the same way over and over again so that a particular way of thinking becomes the default. For example, if we learn that black men are not only male and black, but may be hostile and lazy, our reply to a particular black man could be determined by automatic processes quite beyond our conscious control. We can for example avoid him or treat him poorly without any knowledge of his actual characteristics [8].

Automatic processes are far less flexible than controlled processes and so they are very hard to modify in response to changes in the environment. Automatization typically develops when the same stimulus has to be detected consistently over many trials.

There are some experiments that study the effect of automatization and the hardness of modifiability. For example, Szymura, Slabosz and Orzechowski [13] used the Clock Test to study the speed-accuracy trade-off, automatization and rigidity relationships. In their experiment, subjects had to detect the stimulus (an icon) representing hours on the clock (the dial). There were 40 signals and 40 distracting dials among stimuli. Other icons served as noise (see figure in chapter two). The icon of 4 o'clock was the target to detect for three times. The icon of 5 o'clock was the target to detect for the fourth time. Subjects had 2 minutes to complete the test for each of the four trials. The index of automatization was calculated by the difference in correctness of selectivity mechanism between the third and the first trial and the difference in the number of errors between the third and the first trial (see chapter two). The rigidity index was calculated by the difference in correctness between the third and the fourth trial. Automatization increased the correctness and reduced the errors. Results show also that the higher levels of automatization predict the higher levels of rigidity. Another work [14] had the aim was to ascertain whether automation produces cognitive rigidity. One-hundred and nineteen university students enrolled in the first year of an educational science degree course were invited to complete Moron's Clock test [15] three times in the same version (4 o'clock), and subsequently once in a version which required different responses (5 o'clock). The results indicated that there was a progressive decrease in the number of errors and a progressive increase in speed as the participants completed the three versions of the same task; the participants who best automated performance in visual attention tasks revealed higher levels of cognitive rigidity in the fourth, different version of the test in comparison to participants who automated more slowly. These results were similar to that of McLeod, McLaughlin and Nimmo-Smith [11] which demonstrated that automatic processes may led to stereotypic ability.

Summarizing, the main slips that often involve automatic processing are:

1. Capture error: failure to depart from automatic routine
2. Omission: interruption in routine leads to skipping one or more steps on resumption
3. Perseveration: repeating an already completed process
4. Description: correct action on the wrong object (due to internal description of intended action)
5. Data-Driven error: incoming sensory input overrides intended action (e.g., dialing numbers heard in the environment rather than intended phone number)

6. Associative-Activation error: strong associations lead to wrong automatic behavior (e.g., wrong name, "come in" to doorbell, etc.)
7. Loss-of-activation error: "what am I doing here after entering a room"...
8. Priming
9. Habituation: becoming accustomed to a stimulus such that it no longer draws attention. Subject to conscious control. Not tied to stimulus intensity.
10. Sensory adaptation: a lessening of attention to a stimulus that is not subject to conscious control. Tied to stimulus intensity. Unrelated to number, length, and recency of prior historic exposure (e.g., skin receptor).
11. Dishabituation: change in a familiar stimulus that pulls attention back to processing it.

## CONCLUSION

In this chapter costs and benefits of automatization were analized.

Automatization of cognitive processes has both positive and negative aspects. On the positive side, our ability to respond unconsciously and effortlessly to a range of cognitive and social settings allows us the possibility of speedy responses that are largely appropriate. The negative aspect of automaticity inheres in the lack of flexibility and control that results when we learn too well and are not conscious of doing some tasks. We may make maladaptive or immoral inconscious responses that we then regret or simply fail to notice.

In any case, we know that there is no clear distinction but a gradation between the two processes [16] . Gopher [17] seeks evidence to support the idea that attention management is a skill and that it can be learnt through training. He argues that we would need to show: first, that subjects do actually have the potential to control their allocation of attention, second, that this potential is not always fulfilled, in so far as subjects may fail to maintain control: and last, that with appropriate training, difficulties of control can be overcome. For this reason we can overcome also lack of control of automatic processes.

# REFERENCES

[1]  Saling, L.L., & Phillips, J.G. (2007). Automatic behaviour: Efficient not mindless. *Brain Research Bulletin 73*, 1-20.
[2]  Schneider, W., & Chein, J.M. (2003) . *Controlled & automatic processing: behavior, theory, and biological mechanisms.* Pittsburgh, USA: Department of Psychology, University of Pittsburgh.
[3]  Neely, J.H. (1977). Semantic Primal and retreival from lexical memory: Roles from inhibitionless spreading activation and limited-capacity attention. *Journal of Experimental Psychology: General, 106*, 226 –254.
[4]  Posner, M.I., & Snyder, C.R.R. (1975). Attention and cognitive control. In R. Solso (ed.), *Information Processing and Cognition: The Loyola Symposium* (pp. 550-585). Hillsdale, N.J.: Lawrence Erlbaum Associates.
[5]  Logan, G.D. (1978). Attention in character classification: evidence for the automaticity of component steges. *Journal of Experimental Psychology: General, 107*, 32-63.
[6]  Schneider, W., & Shiffrin, R. M. (1977). Controlled and automatic human information processing: I: Detection, search, and attention. *Psychological Review,84*, 1-66.
[7]  Zbodrof, N. J. & Logan, C. D. (1986). On the autonomy of mental processes. A case study of arithmetic. *Journal of Experimental Psychology: General, 115(2)*, 118-130.
[8]  Weatley, T., & Wegner, D.M. (2001). Automaticity of action, psychology of. *International Encyclopedia of the Social and Behavioural Sciences, 990-993.*
[9]  Parasuraman, R., Hilburn, B., Molloy, R., & Singh, I. (1991). *Adaptive automation and human performance III. Effects of practice on the benefits and costs of automation shifts ( Technical Report CSL-N91-2).* Washington, DC: The Catholic University of America, Cognitive Science Laboratory.
[10] Phillips, J.G. & Triggs, T.J. (2001). Whither automaticity and human performance? In F. Columbus (Ed.), *Advances in Psychology Research IV* (pp. 151-173). Nova Science Publishers.
[11] McLeod, P., McLaughlin, C., & Nimmo Smith, I. (1986). Information encapsulation and automaticity: Evidence from the visual control of finely timed actions. In M.I. Posner & O.S.M. Marin (Eds), *Attention and performance XI*, (pp. 391-406). Hillsdale, NJ: Erbaum.
[12] Carr, T.H., McCauley, C., Sperber, R.D., & Parmalee, C.M. (1982). Words , pictures, and priming: On semantic activation, conscious identification, and

the automaticity of information processing. *Journal of Experimental Psychology: Human Perception and Performance, 8*, 757-777.

[13] Szymura, B., Slabosz, A. & Orzechowski, J., 2001. *Some benefits and costs of the selectivity automatization.* Poster prepared for the 12th Conference of the ESCOP, Edinburgh. 5-8 September 2001.

[14] Fabio, R.A., Pravettoni, G., & Antonietti, A. (2007). Benefici e costi dei processi di automatizzazione dell'attenzione visiva. *Ricerche di psicologia, 3,* 17-29.

[15] Moron, M. (1997). *Unpublished MA Thesis.* Krakow: Jagiellonian University.

[16] Neumann, O. (1984). Automatic processing: A review of recent findings and a plea for an old theory. In W. Printz, & A. Sanders (Eds.), *Cognition and motor processes* (pp. 255-293) . Berlin: Springer.

[17] Gopher, D. (1993), The skill of attention control: Acquisition and execution of attention strategies. In D. Meyer and S. Kornblum (eds.), *Attention and Performance XIV: Synergies in Experimental Psychology, Artificial Intelligence, and Cognitive Neuroscience--A Silver Jubilee,* Cambridge, MA: MIT Press.

# PART II:
# THE INFLUENCE OF AUTOMATIZATION
# ON COMPLEX THINKING

*Chapter 5*

# AUTOMATIZATION: WAY AND DYNAMIC OF ACCESSING TO COMPLEX THINKING

## ABSTRACT

As we seen in the previous chapters, the effects of an extensive practice result in the shift from controlled to automatic processing. For example when learning a new task such as how to play tennis or to drive a car, attention is allocated in order to fulfil task requirements. Performance initially requires controlled processing and is slow, awkward and prone to errors. As training proceeds, performance requires less vigilance, becomes faster and errors decrease, a transformation that can be defined as "automatization". The purpose of this chapter is to analyse how automatization can work. To begin Anderson's theory is considered. In her model the rules of new tasks begin to become proceduralised. This proceduralisation frees space in working memory as the knowledge that was once declarative becomes embedded in procedures which do not need to be retrieved in declarative form. Secondly Gopher's model is considered, then the related Logan's instance theory is presented. In this theory the reduction in RT with practice is explained to occur because subjects employ an alternative strategy of retrieving memory traces left by previous performances ("instances") and directly choosing the retrieved solution without need for calculation. In the last part of the chapter the effects of practice on automatization and access to complex thinking are presented. A model of access to more complex cognitive processes tasks is combined with the catastrophe model to explain the way to access to more complex cognitive processes.

# THE PROCESS OF AUTOMATIZATION

As noted in the first chapter, a number of influential theories proposed in the late 1970s suggested that tasks become "automatized" after they have been executed with sufficient consistent practice [1]. In the initial stages of learning a new task or skill, such as playing the piano, people's performance is usually slow and full of mistakes [2].

As we saw in the second chapter the contrast between automatic and controlled processing was initially studied using extended consistent mapping (CM) training. A consistent mapping task is one in which the response to the stimulus is consistent across extended periods of time (e.g., in a search task, the set of target stimuli is constant throughout the experiment). Under consistent mapping, automatic processes can develop slowly as repeated stimuli are attended to. Although there may be marked performance improvements even within the first few trials [3], full automaticity typically requires hundreds of trials to develop. In varied mapping (VM) training, the relationship of the stimulus to response mapping varies from trial to trial (e.g., in a search task, a stimulus that is assigned a given response on one trial is assigned a different response on the next trial). With varied mapping, the prior and current associations are incompatible, thereby precluding automaticity and the development of an automatic attention response [4].

For example in a chess game, novices repeat the rules to themselves and have to work out the implications of each move one at a time. An expert on the other hand, can rapidly sum up the state of the game and make a good move without seeming to have had a problem to solve at all. Also in a Sudoku game, initially it is very hard remembering the digits and finding the correct position; as playing proceeds, it become easy finding the correct position and remembering many digits.

Automatization is normally understood to mean that a task or operation acquires several properties. One feature is a lack of voluntary control the operation proceeds more or less reflexively given the appropriate stimulus input.

On interrogation the experts may have difficulty in explaining exactly why they made one move rather than another. In contrast to the novice, the experts seems to have poor access to declarative knowledge for the reasons underlying their decision although the expert's performance is much better than that of the novice [5].

Another feature is the lack of interference with other ongoing mental operations. Highly practiced tasks can be performed simultaneously with other tasks without interference (except for structural conflicts such as common reliance on the same effectors, requiring foveation, etc.).

Coming back to the chess game, if television is turned on, the expert can continue the play, but probably the novice will be distracted by it.

In the following part of this chapter theories of automatization will be introduced.

We start with Anderson's theory and Gopher's theory. We presented Anderson'S theory and Gopher'S theory in the first chapter with reference to general ways to deal with automatic and controlled processes. In this chapter we present them again, but with reference to the process of automatization. The chapter proceeds with Logan's istance theory and Pashler's point of view. Afterwards the effect of Practise on  Speed of Processing, on two tasks and on access to complex thinking will be analysed.

## ANDERSON'S THEORY

According to Anderson's theory [6], there are three successive stages of learning involved in the acquisition of cognitive skills. In the beginning, learning involves the collection of relevant facts. So, for example, when learning to play chess, we need to know which moves are legal and which pieces move which way. The novice then applies previous experience in problem solving, to work out which is the best move. However, performance is slow and error prone because of the need to activate and retrieve all relevant knowledge into the working memory. When working memory is overloaded relevant information may be lost and an error result. With more practice, the rules of chess begin to become proceduralised. New productions are formed from the declarative knowledge gained in the initial stages of learning. This proceduralisation frees space in working memory as the knowledge that was once declarative becomes embedded in procedures which do not need to be retrieved in declarative form to be used by the information processing system. So, for example, the rules governing legal moves by different chess pieces are just "known" by the system; the player does not have to keep on retrieving that knowledge into active working memory. The player will also begin to learn that, if a particular configuration of pieces is on the board, making a particular move is likely to produce a good outcome. In the final stages of learning, new procedures are formed from existing productions. This composition of procedures allows complex patterns of IF.. .THEN rules to be compiled, so that the IF side of the production can be made up of several clauses, which will THEN produce one or a series of actions.

Production rules become strengthened with use, and may become so "automatic" that the information within them is no longer available in declarative form. Experts just "know" the answer to problems and may find it extremely difficult to explain why they come to decisions. Once a rule is proceduralised it can be easily applied to novel situations.

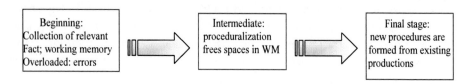

Figure 1. The three stages of learning in Anderson's theory

Coming back to the chess players, Chase and Simon [7] earned out a classic study of chess players. They showed that master chess players could memorise the positions of pieces on a chess board far more quickly than novices, but only when the pieces formed part of a valid game. If the pieces were placed at random, the novices and experts were just the same. It appears that experts perceive board positions in much larger "chunks" than novices. An expert sees the pieces in relational groups whereas the novice sees each piece individually. In terms of production systems the expert has acquired a whole set of productions in which patterns of pieces on the board specify the conditions for making particular moves, which allows information that matches previous experience to be grouped into a coherent whole. Random patterns of pieces do not fit with previous experience and are no easier for the expert than the novice.

Gopher's [8] (1993) experiments on training attentional strategies could be considered in terms of production rules which have aggregated into complex "macro operators". Since productions run off automatically, skill learning can be viewed as procedure learning. As more and more declarative knowledge becomes proceduralised, there is less and less demand on the conscious, strategic processing that is said to be attention demanding. Gopher looks also at how people can learn to improve their attentional skills by training.

One of the tasks used for this training is called the Space Fortress which was designed to present the subject with a complex, dynamic environment within the confines of a well-specified computer game. The players have to control the movements of a space ship as if they were flying it, at the same time as firing missiles, to try to destroy the fortress, but at the same time they must avoid being destroyed themselves. The rules of the game are quite complex and the main aim is to score points. When players first tried the game their first response was usually panic. They felt that the demands of the situation were too high: everything happened too fast; too much happened at once: and the situation seemed to be out of control. This sounds very like our feeling when we first attempt any complex skill, like driving a car. After considerable practice the players began to work out a strategy and performance improved. Without specific training, people would not necessarily work out or adopt an optimal strategy, but Gopher found that if subjects were led through a sequence of emphasis changes for subcomponents of the game, similar to the variable priority method used in POC studies, performance could be improved. Subjects were advised to concentrate on one subcomponent at a time, and respond to the other components only if they could do so without neglecting the component they were to concentrate on. The game remained exactly the same, apart from the introduction of a reward element in that the selected game component received more points (This was to give subjects positive feedback on their success). Otherwise, only the allocation of attentional priorities was altered. Four groups of subjects were studied. The control group were given practice but no specific emphasis training: two groups were given emphasis training on just one task component, mine handling or ship control; and the fourth group of subjects were given emphasis training on both, in alternation. The results showed that the group who had received the double manipulation outperformed all other groups which did not differ from each other. An interesting finding was that although special training finished after six sessions, the improvement in performance continued over the next four sessions to the end of the experiment. This result suggests, as Gopher [8] reports, that after six sessions the double manipulation group "had already internalised their specialised knowledge and gained sufficient control to continue to improve on their own". The application of this kind of training is demonstrated in another study reported by Gopher in which Israeli airforce cadets were given training on a modification of the *Space Fortress* game. Cadets who drop out often do so because they have difficulty coping with the load of a flight task, dividing and controlling attention. In comparison to a control group who were given no training on the game, the experimental cadets who were given double emphasis training, showed a 30% increase in their actual flight performance. The advantage was largest in the manoeuvres requiring integration of several elements. After 18 months there were twice as many graduates in the experimental group as the control group. Gopher points out that the advantage of game training is not because it is similar to actual flying, because real flying is very much more demanding than the game, and the game is not very realistic. What the game does is to train people in the kinds of attentional skills needed in complex situations. Given direct experience with different attentional strategies, performance improves and these skills transfer to new situations and different task demands.

## LONG-TERM WORKING MEMORY AND SKILL

Although productions are stored in long-term memory, they can be run off automatically without any demand on working memory, Ericsson and Kintsch [9] have recently argued that the traditional view of the use of memory in skilled activity needs to include a long-term working memory. They say that current models of memory [10, 11] cannot account for the massively increased demand for information required by skilled task performance. They outline a theory of long-term working memory (LT-WM) which is an extension of skilled memory theory [12] .

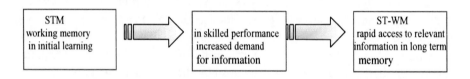

Figure 2. The long-term working memory of Ericsson and Kintsch's theory (1995)

Coming back to the chess players, Chase and Simon [7] earned out a classic study of chess players. The proposal is that in skilled performance, say of chess players, what is needed is rapid access to relevant information in long-term memory. This is achieved by the use of LT-WM in addition to short-term working memory (ST-WM). They suggest that learned memory skills allow experts to use LTM as an extension of ST-WM in areas where they are well practised. LT-WM is basically a set of retrieval structures in LTM. A retrieval structure is a stable organisation made up of many retrieval cues. Load on ST-WM is reduced because rather than all the retrieval cues having to be held there, only the node allowing access to the whole structure need to be available in ST-WM. Thus in skilled performance, all the relevant information stored in LTM is rapidly accessible through the retrieval cue in ST-WM. Indirect evidence for LT-WM was found in a series of experiments by Ericsson and Kintsch, in that a concurrent memory task produced virtually no interference on the working memory of experts. Ericsson and Oliver [13] and Ericsson and Staszewski [14] studied the ability of expert chess players to mentally represent a chess game without the presence of a chess board. Over 40 moves were presented and the chess player's representation of the resulting game position was tested in a form of cued recall task. It was found that his responses were fast and accurate, suggesting a very efficient and accurate memory representation despite the number of moves made, which far exceed the capacity of STWM.

The results suggest that the expert chess player is using this additional LT-WM to maintain and access chess positions. The ability to perforin tasks automatically, therefore, depends on a variety of factors and as we become more expert what we have learnt modifies the way tasks are controlled. In the following part of this chapter we try to understand better how practise acts.

## DOES PRACTISE REDUCES THE DURATION OF COMPONENT STAGES OR ALLOWS TO CARRY OUT CENTRAL OPERATIONS IN PARALLEL?

Recent studies show that practice can dramatically reduce dual-task interference [15, 16, 17, 18]. Thus, the very large interference effects observed with novel tasks (300–400 msec) might overestimate the amount of interference observed between pairs of highly practiced tasks in the real world. In many cases, however, it appears that practice merely reduces stage-durations, without allowing subjects to bypass the processing bottleneck [16, 18]. At the same time, some new evidence suggests that under some conditions practice can eliminate the processing bottleneck entirely [15, 18]. Further work is needed to better define the boundary conditions for these two outcomes.

The reply to this question come from different authors:

## LOGAN'S INSTANCE THEORY

Logan theorized that reductions in RT with practice do not come about from improvements in the speed of executing a basic algorithm used by subjects at low practice levels. Rather, the reduction in RT with practice occurs because subjects employ an alternative strategy of retrieving memory traces left by previous performances ("instances") and directly choosing the retrieved solution without need for calculation.

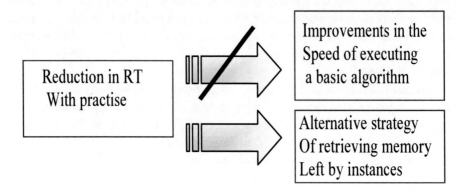

Figure 3. The Logan's model

Logan theorized that the algorithmic process and instance retrieval process operate in parallel in accordance with a "race" model—the first process to finish determines the RT. This theory is called "instance theory". These assumptions imply a learning mechanism that produces a gradual transition from algorithmic processing to memory-based processing.

## PASHLER'S THEORY

Also Pashler [2] discusses recent research on how practice affects the automatization. The key question that the author examines is whether practice merely reduced the duration of component stages of the central bottleneck or allowed subjects to carry out more central operations in parallel on two tasks. Recent evidence suggests that the great bulk of the improvement with practice comes from reducing the duration of central stages, whereas relatively little of the improvement reflects being able to perform central operations on both tasks in parallel.

The question of how practice reduces RTs has been intensively studied in a separate but closely related research area, that of skill learning. Over the past two decades much interest has focussed on the so-called power law of learning. Rosenbloom & Newell [19] proposed this law after observing that in a wide variety of RT tasks the shortening of RT with practice closely followed a power function.

Pashler does not agree with Logan's theory. Because both processes (algorithm-based retrieval and instance retrieval) hypothesized to operate in parallel would seem to be examples of central processes and this theory, as Pashler's point of view appears inconsistent with the conclusions of PRP research [20]. Thus, assessing the validity of this race model is relevant to the goal of providing a unified theory of information processing limitations. An empirical challenge to Logan's race model of improvement with practice has emerged from studies of numerosity judgments about dot patterns. Palmeri [21] reported that judgments in this paradigm improved rapidly with practice, closely following the power law, and data collected using this design initially appeared to be consistent with Logan's model. Rickard [22], however, reanalyzed this data set and argued that although the data showed the usual pattern of a decline in RT over time with a positive second derivative (i.e. practice had diminishing returns over sessions of practice), careful examination showed systematic deviations from a perfect power law fit. Rickard argued that the data more closely fit predictions from his component power law theory. According to this theory, performance during the course of practice reflects a mixture of instance-based and rule-based performance.

The essence of Rickard's model is that on any given trial, subjects perform only the rule-based or the exemplar-based strategy—but not both—and that, over practice, the mixture ratio becomes increasingly shifted toward the exemplar-based strategy. If Rickard's mixture model is correct, contrary to Palmeri's race model, the data can be explained without assuming that subjects can execute both strategies in parallel. Rickard's analysis would be entirely congenial to the findings of the PRP literature suggesting that only one central process can operate at a time.

Palmeri [21] , in a reply to Rickard, argued that more complex versions of the race model can fit the data, but the complexities needed to achieve such fits seem rather uninviting. They include an assumption that the algorithmic process can speed up with practice; it was an important motivation for the Logan model to avoid this assumption. The matter is presently not resolved, and it will be very intriguing if results from future skill-learning studies support or overturn the idea that multiple memory retrieval processes generally cannot, or at least do not, operate in parallel.

In the following part of the chapter we try to understand what changes with practice. Gopher's review has demonstrated that people can operate attentional control and improve with training, but it still seems that it is always "the subject" that is in control, rather than a well-specified cognitive mechanism.

## PRACTICE AND SPEED OF PROCESSING

Several studies have shown that practice produces gradual, continuous increases in processing speed [23, 24, 25, 26] that follow a power law [10, 27, 28, 29]. MacLeod and Dunbar [30] also examined this variable in their study. They continued to train subjects on the shape-naming task with 144 trials per stimulus daily for 20 days. Reaction times showed gradual, progressive improvement with practice.

Another context in which speed of processing was observed is the pattern of interference effects observed in the MacLeod and Dunbar [30] study. In their study interference effect also changed over the course of training on the shape-naming tasks: after 1 day of practice, there was no effect of shape names on color naming. After 5 days of training, however, shapes produced some interference, and after 20 days, there was a large effect. That is, presenting a shape with a name that conflicted with its ink color produced strong interference with the color-naming response.

The reverse pattern of results occurred for the shape-naming task. After 1 session of practice, conflicting ink color interfered with naming the shape, whereas after 20 sessions this no longer occurred. These data suggest that speed of processing and interference effects are continuous in nature and that they are closely related to practice. Furthermore, they indicate that neither speed of processing nor interference effects, alone, can be used reliably to identify processes as controlled or automatic. These observations raise several important questions. The important questions to which MacLeod and Dunbar [30] try to reply are: What is the relationship between processes such as word reading, color naming, and shape naming, and how do their interactions result in the pattern of effects observed? In particular, what kinds of mechanisms can account for continuous changes in both speed of processing and interference effects as a function of practice? Finally, and perhaps most important, how does attention relate to these phenomena?

The purpose of their article is to provide a theoretical framework within which to address these questions. Using the principles of parallel distributed processing (PDP), they describe a model of the Stroop effect in which both speed of processing and interference effects are related to a common, underlying variable that we call *strength of processing*. The model provides a mechanism for three attributes of automaticity. First, it shows how strength varies continuously as a function of practice; second, it shows how the relative strength of two competing processes determines the pattern of interference effects observed; and third, it shows how the strength of a process determines the extent to which it is governed by attention. The model has direct implications for the standard method by which controlled and automatic processes are distinguished.

## PRACTICE AND THE ABILITY TO COMBINE TWO TASKS

People have troubles when they try to combine two tasks. Some tasks could be combined without much difficulty, other tasks are impossible to do together. One explanation for this is that tasks can be combined provided that the mappings between the input and output systems of one task are independent of the mappings between input and output of the other task. If there is crossover between input and output systems required for both tasks, there will be interference. Examples like this were evident in the studies by McLeod and Posner [31] and Shaffer [32]. When tasks can be combined successfully, they seem to be controlled automatically and independently; that is. >, each task shows no evidence of being interfered with by the other and is performed as well in combination as it is alone.

However, when the mappings between the stimuli and their responses are not direct, the tasks interfere with each other and a different kind of control is required, one which requires conscious attention and appears to be of limited capacity. Some tasks which interfere when first combined become independent with enough practice. Also, Spelke, Hirst, and Neisser [33] examined the effect of extended practice on people's ability to combine tasks. They gave two students 85 hours of practice spread over 17 weeks and monitored the ways in which dual-task performance changed over that period.

To begin with, when the students were asked to read stories at the same time as writing to dictation, they found the task combination extremely difficult. Reading rate was very slow and their handwriting was poorly formed. Initially Spelke et al.'s students showed extremely poor performance, but after 6 weeks of extended practice their reading rate had increased: they could comprehend the text; and their handwriting of the dictated words had improved. Tests of memory for the dictated words showed that the students were rarely able to recall any of the words they had written down.

## PRACTICE AND CONTEXT

Also Umiltà [34] (1994) pointed out the effects of an extensive practice result in the shift from controlled to automatic processing. For example when learning a new task such as how to play tennis or to drive a car, attention is allocated in order to fulfil task requirements. Performance initially requires controlled processing and is slow, awkward and prone to errors.

As training proceeds, performance requires less vigilance, becomes faster and errors decrease. This is defined as *automatization.* Automatization can apply to perceptual and motor skills as well as to cognitive processes. Automatized processes can be accomplished simultaneously with other cognitive processes without any interference and task efficiency is optimal.

Job [35] argues that the association of automatic and controlled processes can be understood with reference to the context in which they are activated. As evidenced by Umiltà [34], the context is unusual for the former and usual for the latter. Neuman [36] suggests that practice leads to the development of a skill, which "includes a sensory and, at least during practice, a motor response. After practice the response may remain covert, but is still an attentional response connected to the particular target stimuli. However, even well-practised tasks will display interference if the responses are similar. Tasks may also interfere, according to Neuman, if the initiation of a new response is required; only when there is a continuous stream of information guiding action, as in the Spelke et al. study, can apparent automaticity be found.

## PRACTICE, AUTOMATIZATION AND ACCESS
## TO COMPLEX THINKING

Before starting with the presentation of another effect of automatization it is important to clarify that automaticity and skill are closely related but are not identical. Automatic processes are components of skill, but skill is more than the sum of the automatic components. Automaticity and skill are similar in that both are learned through practice.

In any starting step of a task, initially we use controlled processes of attention to learn and so performance is slow, awkward and prone to errors. We can say that the full amount of our memory load is engaged, we can say also, in other words, that all our cognitive resources are engaged to solve the new learning.

For example we can think of a child that is learning to sum up two numbers. It is very difficult initially for the child to bear in mind the first number, to memorize the second number, to recall the first and to sum up both. It is difficult also to understand that the plus sign means "to add", "to join"... but also "become bigger", "go on"... and so on. So, when the teacher asks him to join the toys of Mary with the toys of Marc, he thinks hardly, he does it slowly and then reaches the result. During his problem solving, if someone asks him something else he makes mistakes in the calculation and forgets the result.

As training proceeds, performance requires less vigilance, becomes faster and errors decrease, a transformation that can be defined as "automatization". With learning, the attentional strategies that once needed control become automatic.

Coming back to the above mentioned child, as learning proceeds, he becomes able to think of the plus sign faster and reaches the result easily. He becomes able to reply also to someone who askS him something else. In other words the child automatizes learning of the plus sign. In the model below we are positioned in the A level, when automatization appears and discharge of cognitive load on A level takes place.

Later the child has to learn how to multiply, or how to sum up and subtract some quantity. If he were totally (or even partially) engaged in the A level, it would be difficult to access to more complex tasks. He can now have access to the execution of subtraction and summing up (B level) thanks to the fact that he assumed the A level as an automatized subroutine.

Again to solve the B level he initially needs the controlled processes of attention and again perfnce is slow, awkward and prone to errors. The full amount of his memory is engaged and all his cognitive resources are engaged to solve the new learning.

As training proceeds, performance requires less vigilance, becomes faster and errors decrease, again we see automatization. In other words, with learning, the attentional strategies that once needed control become automatic. He becomes able to solve problems that need both subtraction and summing up.

Later he has to learn more complex problem solving which requires 3 math operations (C level). The B level that contains the A level becomes again a unique automatized subroutine thanks to the discharge of cognitive load. So now the child can solve these more complex problems. And so on. The infinity symbol that stays at the top of the figure means that there is no limit to the possibility to have access to increasing stages of complex thinking [37]. In effect if we are able to execute complex problem solving, we can go over to more complex ones. If we are able to execute only simple basic discriminations we can learn more complex ones based on the first.

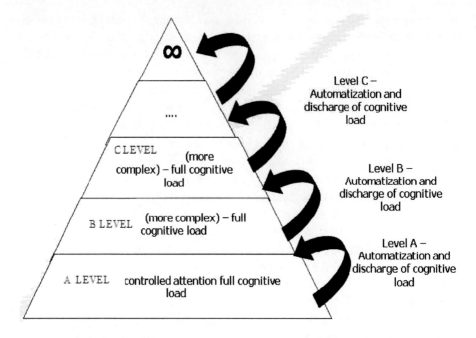

Figure 4. The Fabio's model

Two other questions are related to this model. The first core question is: what happens inside each level, before overcoming it? And the second is: what are the variables linked to skill acquisition?

Starting from the first point, Flor and Dooley [38] explain the learning process that happen inside each level with reference to schemata. Schemata are the outcome of learning. They can be seen as an internal map which facilitate recognition through tags and smaller building-block schemata, and which facilitate actions by linking triggers and actions [39]. Physiologically schemata are distributed electro-chemical networks embedded in connections between neurons. As learning proceeds there may be one or more schemata that evolves; in fact it is possible that schemata compete during the initial stages of learning, and a single dominant schema eventually takes over.

As seen above, in the first chapter, Logan [41] characterizes the process as a progression from a search algorithm schema to a direct retrieval schema. Logan's theory also explains why experts seem to forget all the components steps needed to accomplish complex tasks; the schema developed and used for later performance has gained a magnitude and efficiency due to a reductions in steps.

Subsequently Flor and Dooley [38] explain that the brain's map representing the schema may be simplified. The brain is able to chunk several distinct but interrelated ideas into a unique idea, and this produces access and processing time. Chunking is a very important process and may lead to significant gains in task performance. As seen in the above presented model, assuming the A level as an automatized subroutine means performing a chunking operation.

There are in this case two important explanation on the dynamic of learning to automaticity. The first lies at a neurological level [42] and the second at a meta-cognitive level [43]. From the first view point Mackay et al. [42] argued that practice under consistent conditions simply leads to an increase in the firing between nodes in an existing neural network; from the second view point, Cheng proposes that improvements in performance occur through more efficient restructuring, reordering and reorganization of cognitive tasks.

In order to analyse how the brain can operate under varying conditions Flor and Dooley [38] claim that consistent and changing tasks can be performed in a learning environment and measures of task performance and subsequent analysis should lead to hypotheses concerning which factors account for performance gains. Some mathematical models are used to quantify the relationship between learning environment and task performance. The simplest is the log-linear model [43]:

$$RT (t) = k * t^b$$

where RT (t) is the task response at time t, k and b are empirically determined constants, and t is time (trial). As Flor and Dooley [38] point out the log-linear model assumes rapid initial improvements followed by slow, incremental improvement. It assumes learning occurs through accumulated exposure to stimulus. If one assumes that performance improve only gradually a first, the S-shaped learning curve is appropriate:

$$Ln\, RT (t) = (1/M) \{ A + B\, Ln (t) + C\, Ln (t^2) + D\, \ln (t^3) \}$$

where M, A, B, C, and D are empirically determined. In either case the learning process converges to a point where there is little or no schema development. Dynamically, as Flor and Dooley [38] state, in the learning process there is a point attractor; in general the authors state the first research proposition i.e. that "Performance on a learned task converges to a point attractor" (p. 169).

In statistics convergence is indicated by weak stationarity: that means variance and covariance remain constant and independent of time. Convergence is in part indicated by the lack of divergence or chaotic dynamics. The presence of divergent dynamic is an indication of chaos. The second research proposition is "Initial performance on a learned task exhibits chaotic dynamic" (p. 169).

The output of a chaotic system is point by point unpredictable, but forms a recognizable pattern over time if observed properly. The discovery of chaos leads to a rejection of the random hypothesis.

So, the early stages of the learning processare by a chaotic dynamic, it may be because the brain is searching for optimal chunking patterns. This type of chaotic search has also been found in numerous studies of neuron level activity in which it is known that sensitivity to initial conditions allows amplification of small fluctuations, initial conditions may create and may destroy information.

As performance on the learned task converges, a state of mastery is achieved and so, further exposure to the learning task results in chunking rather than in improvement in performance. Less and less effort is required, and process and action become automatic. Thus chunking may explain why tasks can become automatic. Chunking may tend to follow a model of puntuacted equilibrium, where long period of stasis are interrupted by short period of rapid change [44]. This is similar to the evolutionary dynamic seen in genetic systems and also observed in human societal development. It is similar also to the dynamics of the catastrophe model.

Mathematically the catastrophe model is defined by [45]:

$$Ln\,(RT(t)) = BO + Ln\,(RT\,(t\text{-}1)) + B1 * Q1 + B2 * Q2 * Ln\,(RT(t\text{-}1)) + B3 * Ln\,(RT2(t)) + B4 * Ln\,(RT3(t)) + B5 * Q3$$

where BO through B4 is empirically determined. Q1 is the asymmetry parameter (=t) and Q2 is the bifurcation parameter. This lead the authors to assert the third research proposition that is: A catastrophe model can be used to model the discontinuance dynamics of learning to automaticity.

The second question, related to the model of access to complex thinking is, as Johnson [50] points out, that many skills are too complex to be learned all at once.

Skill acquisition depends on paying attention to the right things at the right time. That is, an important aspect of skilled performance is skilled attending. In many tasks, it is important not only to know what to attend to, but how to attend to it. Complex, dynamic tasks often require performers to divide attention and processing resources among competing, dynamically changing stimuli or task demands, for which priorities must be established and trade-offs made. Important questions in the training of complex skills concern whether we are aware of attentional investments and can control and allocate attentional resources.

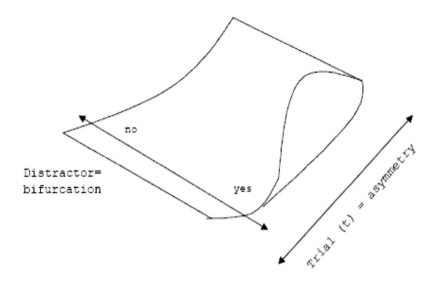

Figure 5. The catastrophe model

Effective training can therefore depend on learning only certain aspects of a skill at a time. For these reasons, methods of decomposing skills for training and then recombining them are needed if effective training programs are to be designed.

The Space Fortress game is a video game developed by researchers to study complex skill acquisition [46], and it is based on task decomposition, an analysis of human information-processing requirements, and the characteristics of expert performance.

Frederiksen and White [47] first identified the hierarchical relationships between skill and knowledge components that allow the progression from novice to expert performance and then used this task decomposition to construct training activities for the component processes as well as their integration. A comparison of the performance of a group who received componential training and a control group who practiced the Space Fortress game showed an initial deficit for the componential-training group when first transferred to whole-game performance. However, the componential-training group quickly overtook the whole-game training group, suggesting that, after some initial integration of learned skills during their first experience with the whole game, the specific knowledge and heuristics taught in the componential training had benefited learning.

In general, part-task training, such as that used by Frederiksen and White [47], has been shown to be an effective method of training difficult tasks or tasks with independent components [48, 49]. Several methods of part-task training have been developed and evaluated. If a task consists of components with clear starting and stopping points, it can simply be segmented into the different components. If the last step in a segmented task is practiced first, with earlier components added later, the procedure is called backward chaining. Whether backward chaining is more effective than forward chaining, in which segments are trained sequentially, starting with the first one, will depend on the type of feedback needed for performance.

As Johnson [50] points out for complex tasks in which the initial steps are far removed from the goal, there might be a benefit for backward chaining because this begins by emphasizing the steps closest to the goal. When feedback from one component influences performance on the next, forward chaining might be more effective [49]. Marmie and Healy [51] showed that the benefits of parttask training using a segmentation and backward-chaining strategy can show long-lasting effects in a simulated tankgunnery task. In the relevant experiment, participants practiced either the whole task (searching for a target, sighting it, and firing) or, for several sessions, only the sighting and firing components. Performance in whole-task retention sessions given immediately after training or one month later showed no difference between the groups in overall performance (proportion of kills) or in time to identify the target. However, the part-task training group, which was able to devote more resources to the sighting and firing components of the task during training, showed a long-lasting benefit in time to fire.

If different task components are performed in parallel, it is not possible to segment them. In this case, we speak of fractionation of the task. This involves practicing some components, such as perceptual skills, in isolation and then combining them with other aspects of the task, such as making responses. It has been argued that fractionation can only be effective if there is relatively little time sharing or interdependence between the components [52]. In some cases, such as when multiple-task components must be carried out in parallel, the demands imposed by the need to recombine the separate skills counteract any benefits of part-task training. However, the view that part-task training is ineffective for tasks that must be time shared may be overly pessimistic.

## AUTOMATICITY AND TRAINING

Attentional strategies can be trained, but to what extent can people be trained to operate without attention? Many complex tasks can only be performed because some task components have become automatized, thus freeing up resources for other components. Several researchers have shown that training in tasks similar to visual search can lead to automatic processing. Such training has been used successfully with air traffic controllers to promote automatic processing of some perceptual information, such as the distances between aircraft, and indications of certain maneuvers, such as the start of turns [53]. Shebilske, Goettl, and Regian [54] have developed a framework for training that emphasizes the development of automaticity in task components. They suggest that by determining the components for which automaticity does not develop, one succeeds in identifying those components that play a controlling, or executive, role in the performance of a task.

## CONCLUSION

In this chapter theories about automatization were presented. A model and an attempt to understand if automatization can be the way to access to more complex cognitive processes was analysed.

The first paradigm was the Anderson model. In her model with practice, the rules of new tasks begin to become proceduralised. New productions are formed from the declarative knowledge gained in the initial stages of learning. This proceduralisation frees space in working memory as the knowledge that was once declarative becomes embedded in procedures which do not need to be retrieved in declarative form to be used by the information processing system.

In Gopher's [8] point of view, experiments on training attentional strategies could be considered in terms of production rules which have aggregated into complex "macro operators". Since productions run off automatically, skill learning can be viewed as procedure learning. As more and more declarative knowledge becomes proceduralised there is less and less demand on the conscious, strategic processing that is said to be attention demanding. Gopher looks also at how people can learn to improve their attentional skills by training.

What the game does is to train people in the kinds of attentional skills needed in complex situations. Given direct experience with different attentional strategies, performance improves and these skills transfer to new situations and different task demands.

In Logan's instance theory it is theorized that reductions in RT with practice do not come about from improvements in the speed of executing a basic algorithm used by subjects at low practice levels. Rather, the reduction in RT with practice occurs because subjects employ an alternative strategy of retrieving memory traces left by previous performances ("instances") and directly choosing the retrieved solution without need for calculation.

Also Pashler [2] discusses recent research on how practice affects the automatization. The key question that the author examines is whether practice merely reduced the duration of component stages of the central bottleneck or allowed subjects to carry out more central operations in parallel on two tasks. Recent evidence suggests that the great bulk of the improvement with practice comes from reducing the duration of central stages, whereas relatively little of the improvement reflects being able to perform central operations on both tasks in parallel.

The question of how practice reduces RTs has been intensively studied in a separate but closely related research area, that of skill learning.

Neuman [36] suggests that practice leads to the development of a skill, which includes a sensory and, at least during practice, a motor response. After practice the response may remain covert, but is still an attentional response connected to the particular target stimuli. However, even well-practised tasks will display interference if the responses are similar. Tasks may also interfere, according to Neuman, if the initiation of a new response is required; only when there is a continuous stream of information guiding action, as in the Spelke et al. study, can apparent automaticity be found.

In the last part of the chapter the effect of practice on automatization and access to complex thinking was presented.

The core assumption is that as training proceeds, performance requires less vigilance, becomes faster and errors decrease and we see automatization. With learning, the attentional strategies that once needed control become automatic. The subject becomes able to solve more complex problems. Thanks to discharge of cognitive load that can be engaged to more complex tasks.

# REFERENCES

[1]    Schneider, W., & Shiffrin, R. M. (1977). Controlled and automatic human information processing:1. Detection search and attention. *Psichological Review, 84*, 1-66.

[2]    Pashler, H. (2001). Involuntary orienting to flashing distracters in delayed search. In C.L. Folk & B. Gibson(Eds). *Attraction, distraction and action: multiple perspectives on attentional capture. Advances in psychology.* Elsevier.

[3]    Logan, G.D. (1992). Attention and Preattention in Theories of Automaticity. *The American Journal of Psychology, 105, 2*, 317-339.

[4]    Schneider, W., & Chein, J.M. (2003) . *Controlled & automatic processing: behavior, theory, and biological mechanisms.* Pittsburgh, USA: Department of Psychology, University of Pittsburgh.

[5]    Styles, E. A. (2007). *The psychology of attention.* London: The Taylor & Francis e-Library.

[6]    Anderson. J.R. (1983). *The architecture of cognition.* Cambridge, MA: Harvard University Press.

[7]    Chase, W.G., & Simon, H.A. (1973). Perception in chess. *Cognitive Psychology, 4*, 55-81.

[8]    Gopher, D. (1993). The skill of attentional control: Acquisition and execution of attentional strategies. In S. Kornblum, & D.E. Meyer (Eds.), *Attention andperformanceXIV: Synergies in experimental psychology, artificial intelligence and cognitive neuroscience.* Cambridge, NLA: MIT Press.

[9]    Ericsson, K.A., & Kintsch, W. (1995). Long-term working memory. *Psychological Review, 102,* 211-245.

[10]   Anderson,S.R. (1982). Acquisition of a cognitive skill. *Psychological Review,89,* 369-406.

[11]   Baddeley. A.D. (1986). *Working memory.* Oxford: Oxford University'Press.

[12]   Chase, W.G. & Ericsson, K.A. (1982). Skill and working memory.In G.H. Bower (Ed.). *The psychology- of learning and motivation* (Vol.16, pp. 1-58). New York: Academic Press.

[13]   Ericsson, K.A., & Oliver, W. (1984, November). *Skilled memory in blindfold chess: Paper presented at the annual meeting of the Psychonomic Society.* San Antonio,TX.

[14]   Ericsson. K.A. & Staszewski. J. (1989). Skilled memory and expertise: Mechanisms of exceptional performance. In D.Klalir & K.Kotovsky (Eds.).

*Complex information processing: The impact of Herbert A.Simon* (pp. 235-267). Hillsdale, NJ: Lawrence Erlbaum Associates Inc.

[15] Hazeltine, E., Teague, D., & Ivry, R.B. (2002). Simultaneous dualtask performance reveals parallel response selection after practice. *Journal of Experimental Psychology: Human Perception and Performance, 28,(3),* 527–545.

[16] Ruthruff, E., Van Selst, M., Johnston, J. C., & Remington, R. W. (2006). How does practice reduce dual-task interference: Integration, automatization, or simply stage-shortening? *Psychological Research, 70,* 125-142.

[17] Schumacher, E. H., Seymour, T. L., Glass, J. M., Kieras, D. E., & Meyer, D. E. (2001). Virtually perfect time sharing in dual-task performance: Uncorking the central attentional bottleneck. *Psychological Science, 12,* 101–108.

[18] Van Selst, M., Ruthruff, E., & Johnston, J. C. (1999). Can practice eliminate the psychological refractory period effect? *Journal of Experimental Psychology: Human Perception and Performance, 25,* 1268–1283.

[19] Newell, A., & Rosenbloom, P. S. (1987). An architecture for general intelligence. *Artificial Intelligence, 33,* 1-64

[20] Pashler , H. & Jonston, J. C. (1998). Attentional limitation in dual –task performance. In Pashler, H.(Ed), *Attention Psycholgy Press* (edition, pp. 155-189). Erlbaum, UK: Taylor & Francis.

[21] Palmeri, T.J. (1999). Theories of automaticity and the power law of practice. *Journal of Experimental Psychology: Learning, Memory, and Cognition, 25,* 543–551.

[22] Rickard, T. C. (1999). A CMPL alternative account of practice effects in numerosità judgment tasks. *Journal of Experimental Psychology: Learning, Memory, and Cognition, 25,* 532-542.

[23] Blackburn, J. M. (1936). Acquisition of Skill: An Analysis of Learning Curves. *IHRB Report , 73.*

[24] Bryan, W. L., & Harter, N. (1899). Studies of the telegraphic language. The acquisition of a hierarchy of habits. *Psychological Review, 6,* 345-375.

[25] Logan, G. D. (1979). On the use of a concurrent memory load to measure attention and automaticity. *Journal of Experimental Psychology: Human Perception and Performance, 5,* 189-207.

[26] Shiffrin, R. M., & Schneider, W. (1977). Controlled and automatic human information processing: II: Perceptual learning, automatic attending, and a general theory. *Psychological Review, 84,* 127-190.

[27]  Kolers, P.A. (1976). Reading a year later. *Journal of Experimental. Psychology:Human Learning and Memory, 2* , 8-10.

[28]  Logan, G. D. (1988). Toward an instance theory of auto matization..*Psychological Review*, *95*, 492-527.

[29]  Newell, A., & Rosenbloom, P. S. ( 1981). Mechanisms of skill acquisition and the law of practice. In J. R. Anderson (Ed.), *Cognitive skills and their acquisition* (pp. 1-55). Hillsdale, NJ: Erlbaum.

[30]  MacLeod, CM. & Dunbar, K. (1988). Training and Stroop-like interference: Evidence for a continuum of autoniaticity. *Journal of Experimental Psychology: Learning, Memory and Cognition, 14,* 137-154.

[31]  McLeod, P., & Posner, M. I. (1984). Privileged loops from percept to act. In H. Bouma & D. G. Bouwhuis (Eds.), *Attention and performance X: Control of language processes* (pp. 55–66). London: Erlbaum.

[32]  Shaffer, L. H. (1975). Multiple attention in continuous verbal tasks. In P. M. A. Rabbitt & S. Dornic (Eds.), *Attention and performance V* (pp.157–167). New York: Academic Press.

[33]  Spelke, E., Hirst, W., & Neisser, U. (1976). Skills of divided attention. *Cognition, 4,* 215-230.

[34]  Umiltà, C., Moscovitch, M. (1994). *Attention and performance XV: Consciuos and nonconsious information processing.* Cambridge: MIT Press.

[35]  Job, R. (1998). I processi cognitivi: modelli e ricerca in psicologia. Roma: Carocci ed.

[36]  Neuman, O. (1984). Automatic processing: A review of recent findings and a plea for an old theory. In Printz,W., & Sanders, A. (Eds.). *Cognition and motor processes.* Berlin: Springer.

[37]  Fabio, R.A. (2005). Dynamic assessment of intelligence is a better reply to adaptive behaviour and cognitive plasticity, *Journal of General Psychology*, 2005, 132, 41-64

[38]  Flor, R., & Dooley, K. (1999). The Dynamics of Learning to Automaticity. *Noetic Journal, 2,* 168-173.

[39]  Holland, J. (1995). *Hidden Order.* Reading, Mass: Addison-Wesley.

[40]  Gallistel, W. (1993). *The Organization of Learning.* Cambridge, Mass: MIT Press.

[41]  Logan, G. (1990). Repetition priming and automaticity. *Cognitive Psychology*, 22, 1-35.

[42]  Mackay, W.A., & Crammond, D.J. (1987) Neuronal correlates in posterior parietal lobe of the expectation of events. *Behavioural Brain Research*, 24, 167-169.

[43] Badiru, A. (1992). Computation survey of univariate and multivariate learning curve models. IEEE Transactions on Engineering Management 39(2): 176-188.

[44] Gould, S. (1980). Is a new and general theory of evolution emerging? Paleobiology 6:119-130.

[45] Guastello, S. (1995). Chaos, Catastrophes, and Human Affairs. Mahwah, NJ: Erlbaum.

[46] Mané, A.M., & Donchin, E. (1989). The Space Fortress game. Acta Psychologica, 71, 17-22.

[47] Frederiksen, S. R., & White, B. Y. (1989). An approach to training based upon prinpled task decomposition. ACTA Psicological , 71,89-146.

[48] Holding, D. H. (1965). Principles of training. Oxford, UK: Pergamon Press.

[49] Wightman, D. C., & Linter, G. (1985). Part-task training strategie for tracking and manual control. Hum . Factor, 27,267-283.

[50] Johnson, A. (2003). Procedural Memory and Skill Acquisition. In A. F. Healy, R.W. Proctor & I.B. Weiner, Handbook of Psychology (pp. 499-523). John Wiley & Sons, Inc.

[51] Marmie, W. R., & Healy, A. F. (1995). The long-term retention of a complex skill. In A. F. Healy & L. E. Bourne, Jr. (Eds.), Learning and memory of knowledge and skills: Durability and specificity (pp. 30–65). Thousand Oaks, CA: Sage.

[52] Schneider,W., & Detweiler, M. (1988). The role of practice in dualtask performance: Toward workload modeling in a connectionist/control architecture. Human Factors, 30, 539–566.

[53] Schneider, W., Vidulich, M., & Yeh, Y.Y. (1982). Training spatial skills for air-traffic control. Proceedings of the Human Factors Society 26th Annual Meeting (10–14). Santa Monica, CA: Human Factors Society.

[54] Shebilske, W., Goettl, B., & Regian, J. W. (1999). Executive control of automatic processes as complex skills develop in laboratory and applied settings. In D. Gopher & A. Koriat (Eds.), Attentionand performance: Vol. 17. Cognitive regulation of performance: Interaction of theory and application (pp. 401–432). Cambridge, MA: MIT Press.

*Chapter 6*

# THE ROLE OF AUTOMATIZATION
# IN SOCIAL SETTINGS

## ABSTRACT

There are several areas of social psychological research for which issues of control and automaticity have special relevance. Attaining an understanding of a person is a seriously important activity in social life. Control and automatic processes are both involved in this enterprise, but the general trend in this area of research has been to examine the degree to which social cognition proceeds automatically- against the background assumption that the balance of the processes involved include the exercise of conscious control. The purpose of this chapter is to present some operational implications of automatic and controlled processes in the field of social cognition. Initially the role of automatization on attitude is presented; then the reflective-reflexive model based in neurocognitive systems and the techniques of neuroimaging that can make great contributions to the understanding of judgment and decision-making are presented. Afterwards the role of automatization on social attribution and stereotyping is explained. Finally the role of automatization on emotions is presented, particularly the "modal model" of emotion that is important as an initial framework for the field. Using this framework, emotion researchers have developed methods that have yielded a large number of empirical findings.

## THE ROLE OF AUTOMATIZATION ON ATTITUDE

An attitude is a hypothetical construct that represents an individual's degree of like or dislike for an item. Attitudes are generally positive or negative views of a person, place, thing, or event-- this is often referred to as the attitude object.

Breckler and Wiggins (1992) define attitudes as "mental and neural representations, organized through experience, exerting a directive or dynamic influence on behavior" (p. 409). Attitudes and attitude objects are functions of cognitive, affective and conative components. Attitudes are part of the brain's associative networks, the spider-like structures residing in long term memory (Higgins, 1986) that consist of affective and cognitive nodes linked through associative pathways (Anderson, 1983; Fazio, 1986). These nodes contain affective, cognitive, and behavioral components (Eagly & Chaiken, 1995).

Anderson (1983) suggests that the inter-structural composition of an associative network can be altered by the activation of a single node. Thus, by activating an affective or emotion node, attitude change may be possible, though affective and cognitive components tend to be intertwined. In primarily affective networks, it is more difficult to produce cognitive counterarguments in the resistance to persuasion and attitude change (Eagly & Chaiken, 1995).

Wegner and Barg (2000) outlined that attitudes are formed just because the person is exposed to the novel attitude object repeatedly over time (Zajonc. 1968). So, we can consider them to have developed automatically.

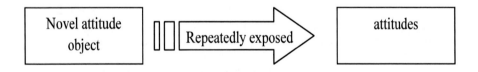

Figure 1. The Wegner and Barg's view

This mere exposure effect appears to be due to a build up in strength of the representation of the novel object with repeated exposure to it that increases the ease of perceiving the object (Gordon & Holyoak, 1983). That the mere exposure effect does not require conscious involvement to occur is indicated by the often replicated finding by Kunst-Wilson and Zajonc (1980) that the effect occurs even with repeated subliminal presentation of novel stimuli. Findings of Monahan, Murphy & Zajonc (2002) suggest also that affect generated by subliminal repeated exposure is sufficiently diffuse to influence ratings of unrelated stimuli and mood.

With reference to earlier research having to do with automatic attitude formation and self- association, the researchers sought to show that the positive attitude toward the object is generated as a result of the subjects' positive feelings about themselves. To demonstrate how easily an association can be created between a consumer and an object, Perkins, Forehand and Greenwald (2007) asked participants to complete a simple categorization test on a computer, pairing words that represent the self, such as "my," "mine," and "me" with a trivial target object, specifically an analog or digital clock. One group of subjects was meant to identify with the analog clocks and the other with digital clocks. The analog clock subjects were told to press the letter "d" on the keyboard if words related to analog clocks or "self" appeared on the monitor, and the letter "k" if words related to digital clocks or "other" appeared on the screen. Participants meant to associate with digital clocks completed categorizations with "self" and "digital" sharing a response. In a second experiment, they replaced the clock images with a series of fictitious individual brand names. After manipulating associations between the subjects and objects, the researchers utilized the Implicit Association test (IAT). The IAT is an experimental method within social psychology designed to measure the strength of automatic association between mental representations of objects (concepts) in memory. The IAT requires the rapid categorization of various stimulus objects, such that easier pairings (and faster responses) are interpreted as being more strongly associated in memory than more difficult pairings (slower responses). The aim of Perkins, Forehand and Greenwald (2007) was to determine if these links to the subjects generated positive attitudes toward these objects. Their earlier studies on the unconscious effects of celebrity voiceovers on brand attitude were among the first to apply this computer-based categorization task to consumer behaviour. They found that the creation of even trivial associations between an individual and an object prompted the individual to identify with and feel positive toward that object.

Another automatic source of attitude formation is via classical conditioning: the association of the novel attitude object with another object or event that already has a positive or negative valence.

Novel attitude object stimuli were paired with subliminal emotional facial expressions, and subsequently expressed attitudes toward these novel objects were in line with the valence of the UCS (facial expressions) associated with them during the study phase of the experiment.

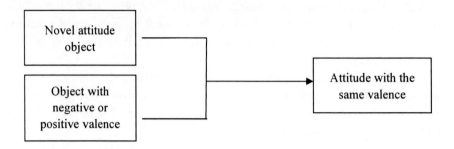

Figure 2. The formation of attitude

A form of automatic attitude formation happens in the finding of Cacioppo, Priester, and Berntson (1993) that muscular feedback influences attitude formation. They discover that attitude formation is preconsciously automatic (and a case of multitasking) because the participants in the experiment were not aware of any relation between their arm positions and their feelings about the novel attitude objects.

Wegner and Barg (2000) point out also Models of Attitude Change. They explain different models: Chaiken's (1980) heuristic-systematic model (HSM), Elaboration-Likelihood Model (ELM) and Fazio's (1986, 1990)' Automatic Attitude Activation model.

With reference to the first, systematic corresponds to an effortful consideration of the arguments. Heuristic processing, on the other hand, makes use of simple decision rules (e.g., "length equals strength" of JA argument) which enable decisions to be made as to accept or reject the persuasive attempt without effortful consideration and weighing of the arguments themselves.

The Elaboration-Likelihood Model (ELM) of persuasive message processing (Petty & Cacioppo, 1984) also distinguishes between two routes to persuasion; a "central" route in which the quality and logic of the arguments themselves are the basis for the attitude change, and a "peripheral" route in which other features of the persuasion situation are the basis.

Fazio (1986) thinks that automatic processing is involved in all aspects of attitude functioning, from formation to change processes to the effect of attitude on behavior. The growing body of evidence of automaticity in these areas is conceptually related to the growing evidence of automaticity in affective information processing more generally, especially for models of attitudes that focus particularly on their evaluative dimension.

Wegner and Barg (2000) conclude that models of persuasion taking into account such dual processes bear some similarity to the distinction between control and automatic processes but also differ from it in important ways.

## THE ROLE OF AUTOMATIZATION ON SOCIAL JUDGMENT

**Social judgment** refers to how we perceive people, how we form impressions about them and how we think about social things.

Lieberman (2004) points out that at every turn and at each moment in our daily lives we are making countless implicit judgments and decisions that allow us to seamlessly make sense of and navigate our social world. We intuitively make sense of the nonverbal messages in the environment and often reciprocate appropriately without any effort (Ambady & Rosenthal, 1993; Chen & Bargh, 1999; Word, Zanna & Cooper, 1974); automatically judge objects as more likeable based on previous exposure or their position in a display (Nisbett & Wilson, 1977; Zajonc, 1968); spontaneously make sense of behavior in terms of intentions and traits (Gilbert, 1989; Heider & Simmel, 1944; Winter & Uleman, 1984); and decide whether to help strangers based merely on the syntax of the request without careful consideration (Langer, Blank & Chanowitz, 1978).

As long as the judgments to be made address familiar stimuli that are functioning in the way we are accustomed, our judgments can usually proceed automatically without ever becoming a focus of attention. However, when our expectations are violated, doubt and ambiguity ensue followed quickly by more explicit decision-making processes.

Lieberman, Gaunt, Gilbert, & Trope (2002) point out that when reflexive processes fail, *reflective* processes are recruited to deal with circumstances that are exceptions to our implicit expectations. As Lieberman et al. outline these terms are defined functionally and neurally, and not just in terms of resistance to cognitive load and other standard measures of automaticity. As we saw in the first chapter dual-process theories typically propose that the occurrence of controlled processing depends on the availability of cognitive resources and the motivation to be accurate. The reflection model, taking its cue from cybernetic control models (Carver & Scheier, 1981; Miller, Galanter, & Pribram, 1960; Wiener, 1948), suggests that in addition to motivation and resources, the occurrence of reflective processes is determined by the success or failure of reflexive processes.

On social judgments Wegner and Barg (2007) present four privileged types of Access to the Judgment Process: information related to the self; information that is frequently experienced; information about negatively valued social behavior; and social category information.

Self-relevant information chronically attracts our attention, the most famous example being our own name-a phenomenon known as the "cocktail party effect" (Cherry, 1953). This effect refers to the ability to focus one's listening attention on a single talker among a mixture of conversations and background noises, ignoring other conversations. This effect reveals one of the surprising abilities of our auditory system, which enables us to talk in a noisy place.

The cocktail party effect can occur both when we are paying attention to one of the sounds around us and when it is invoked by a stimulus which grabs our attention suddenly. For example, when we are talking with our friend in a crowded party, we still can listen and understand what our friend says even if the place is very noisy, and can simultaneously ignore what another nearby person is saying. Then if someone over the other side of the party room calls out our name suddenly, we also notice that sound and respond to it immediately. The hearing reaches a noise suppression from 9 to 15 dB, i.e., the acoustic source, on which humans concentrate, seems to be three times louder than the ambient noise. A microphone recording in comparison will show the big difference. It is as if we have sensitive antennae that pick up self-relevant information even when we are not intending to pick it up.

Frequently attended information is the second kind of "most favored information" for social judgment. Higgins, King, and Mavin (1982) found that in reading about the behaviors of another person, people attended to and later remembered certain kinds of behaviour more than others. Presumably, those that came to mind first, without prompting by semantic or other associative relations with other dimensions, were those that the individual used very frequently in thinking about other people (see also Wegner, 1977). Higgins et al. (1982) termed these chronically accessible trait constructs, in that they led to the pickup of relevant behavioral information without priming or recent use.

A third general source of automatic attention responses is negative social behaviour, including negative emotional expressions (Fiske. 1980: Hansen & Hansen, 1988; Pratto & John, 1991). People seem to be especially vigilant about negative or potentially threatening social information (Wegner & Vallacher. 1977).

Features that signal a person's social category membership represent a fourth kind of "most favored information" that has privileged access to the mind. Easily discriminable personal features-especially the "big three" of gender, Race, and age-tend to activate preconsciously the categories or stereotypes associated with them (e.g., Bargh, 1994; Brewer, 1988; Fiske & Neuberg, 1990; Macrae, Stangor,& Milne, 1994).

With reference to chapter 3 of this book dealing with neurocognitive systems involved in automatic and controlled processes, Lieberman (2004) goes more in depth and shows two neurocognitive systems involved in reflective and reflexive processing on social judgment. On the one hand, these two systems correspond to a cognitive processing dichotomy that have been around for a generation or more: automatic vs. controlled and implicit vs. explicit. At the same time, these old dichotomies are limited in their ability to provide adequate treatment to the positive contributions of each half of the dichotomy. The neural correlates associated with these two types of processes are the X-system (for the X in reflexive) and the C-system (for the C in reflective). Functionally, the X-system is responsible for linking affect and social meaning to currently represented stimuli regardless of whether those stimuli are activated bottom-up as a result of ongoing perception or top-down as the contents of working memory in the form of goals, explicit thought, or retrieved memories. These links usually reflect conditioning between the various features of a stimulus or between the stimulus and the outcomes for which the stimulus is a cue. The former ('stimulus-stimulus' associations) might include implicit personality theories, stereotypes, and other forms of categorical cognition in which various characteristics, traits, or attributes are believed to co-occur.

The latter ('stimulus-outcome' associations) generally refer to affective processes, in which one cue (e.g., an angry expression) indicates that one's goals are about the be advanced or thwarted. These affective processes have long been thought to prepare the individual to act on the basis of affective judgment and thus these processes are assumed to link directly to motor systems in the brain (Frijda, 1986; LeDoux, 1996; Rolls, 1999).

The three neural structures associated with the X-system are the amygdala, basal ganglia and lateral temporal cortex. The C-system is designed to sense the floundering of the X-system and intervenes when appropriate. Of course, in the modern world the C-system is activated much of the time regardless of the X-system's preparedness. That is to say, while the C-system may have evolved to come to the X-system's rescue, the C-system has clearly taken on a life of its own in a world in which nearly every external cue is designed to evoke some degree of C-system processing. Moreover, the rationalist tradition of western society looks down upon the use of intuition (Bruner, 1957; Haidt, 2001; Hogarth,2001; Lieberman, 2000a) and consequently people may tend to rely on C system processing even when X-system is implied.

One of the basic principles of automaticity contends that genuinely automatic processes cannot be disrupted by controlled processes (Bargh, 1999). Controlled processes may frequently set automatic processes in motion, but the ability to run to completion once started is one of the hallmarks of automaticity theory dating back to James (1890). A number of judgment and decision making studies conducted by Wilson and colleagues (Wilson, Dunn, Kraft, & Lisle, 1989; Wilson et al., 1993) highlight a possible exception to this rule. In Wilson's work, participants are required to generate careful introspective accounts of choices that would otherwise be made intuitively.

Using a variety of outcome criteria, Wilson has found that introspection leads to poorer decisions. In one study (Wilson et al., 1993), participants were asked to provide ratings of five posters, some of which were artistic prints by Van Gogh and Monet and others were humorous posters with captions. Only five percent of control participants preferred the humorous posters, while 36% of participants asked to introspect on the basis for their preference chose the humorous poster. Additionally, participants were allowed to take a copy of their preferred print home with them. When contacted weeks later, participants that had been in the introspection condition expressed less satisfaction with their earlier choice than did the control participants. Thus, introspecting on the reasons for our preferences changes our preferences temporarily, leading to outcomes that are less satisfactory in the long run.

Lieberman points out that by focusing on the neural basis of these systems, links can be made to the known computational characteristics of these systems and these characteristics provide us with important clues as to why the two systems provide us with the outputs they do. Furthermore, current operationalizations of automaticity and control make it difficult to identify anything but the relative contributions of each system, rather than the absolute contributions of each. Finally, this operationalization assumes that the effects of automatic and controlled processes add and subtract linearly without interaction effects. Neuroimaging allows the study of the ongoing interactions between the two systems.

## THE ROLE OF AUTOMATIZATION
## ON ATTRIBUTION AND STEREOTYPING

In social psychology, attribution refers to how individuals explain causes of events, other's behavior, and their own behavior. The two main types of attributions are internal and external attributions. When an internal attribution is made, the cause of the given behavior is assigned to the individual's personality, attitudes, character, or disposition. When an external attribution is made, the cause of the given behavior is assigned to the situation in which the behavior was seen. The individual producing the behavior did so because of the surrounding environment or the social situation. These two types of attribution lead to very different perceptions of the individual engaging in a behavior. Personal is Internal and Situational is external.

With reference to stereotyping, it appears when a preconceived idea that attributes certain characteristics (in general) to all the members of class or set. Stereotypes often form the basis of prejudice and are usually employed to explain real or imaginary differences due to race, gender, religion, ethnicity, socio-economic class, disability, occupation, etc. Stereotypes are forms of social consensus rather than individual judgments. Stereotypes are sometimes formed by a previous illusory correlation, a false association between two variables that are loosely correlated if correlated at all.

To a certain extent, categorizing people quickly and efficiently in terms of their group membership is adaptive and defensible in that we cannot possibly attend and individuate everyone we encounter. Macrae, Milne, and Bodenhausen (1993) have found that stereotypes do allow for more efficient processing of information about people, in that less attentional capacity is needed and can thus be devoted to other, goal-relevant tasks. Dijksterhuis and van Knippenberg (1996a) provide evidence suggesting that stereotyping is inevitable. The automatic stereotype activation depends on the strength of the association between the representation of the group (including distinguishing group features) and the representation of the group stereotype in memory. While for many stereotypes this connection may be so frequently used by most people that it becomes automatic for the average person, for other stereotypes that are less implicitly assumed by members of the culture, this connection may be more tenuous.

Pratto and Bargh (1991) found that gender stereotypes become active to influence judgments about a target person even under information overload conditions; that is efficiently (see also Macrae et al., 1993). One might expect this connection between representation of a group and its stereotypic trait concepts to vary strength as a function of the prejudice level of the individual.

The subliminal presentation of stimuli related to the stereotype activated the entire stereotype, including content not presented as priming stimuli such as "hostile," for all participants regardless of their responses on the racism scale. Stereotype activation was evidenced by more hostile ratings of a target person in a subsequent impression formation task by those participants exposed to the stereotype- relevant stimuli. Bargh, Chen, and Burrows (1996) recently found that subliminal presentation of African-American faces to white male participants resulted in increases in the participant's own hostile behavior- a behavioral effect of automatic stereotype activation- and again this effect was not moderated by participants' Modern Racism scores.

## THE ROLE OF AUTOMATIZATION ON EMOTION EXPERIENCE

An emotion is a mental and physiological state associated with a wide variety of feelings, thoughts, and behaviors. Emotions are subjective experiences, or experienced from an individual point of view. Emotion experience permeates our conscious life. Whether subtle or overwhelming, expressed and shared, or hidden and suffocated, feelings render consciousness personally relevant.

Emotions are also assumed to be primitive, automatic, animalistic entities dwelling within us that the more developed human parts of our minds come to know about and control. Emotional states so happen to us automatically. The idea that emotion onset is automatic comes from a variety of literatures, most of which point to the "basicness" of emotional expression and behavior. Emotion seems basic in view of the similarity of human emotional behavior to animal emotional behavior (Andrew, 1963), the early development of emotional responses (Emde 1984) and processes of emotion imitation (Haviland & Lelwica, 1987), the evolutionary primitiveness of some of the brain centers that govern emotion (MacLean, 1993), and the cross-cultural similarity of emotion expressions (Ekman, 1992).

In this view, our emotions are rarely, if ever, the product of controlled, deliberate, and conscious thought. Although it is possible to "think ourselves" into an emotional state, controlled processes typically serve to control, rather than to elicit, emotional responses.

Barret, Ochsner and Gross (2006) state that there are some basic scientific approaches to emotion. Dual-process models pervade contemporary psychology (e.g., Barrett, Tugade, & Engle, 2004; Chaiken & Trope, 1999; Devine, 1989; Gilbert, 1991, 1998; Power & Dalgleish, 1997; Schacter, 1997; Sloman, 1996; Smith & DeCoster, 2000; Trope, 1986). A central tenet of such models is that behaviour is determined by the interplay of automatic and controlled processing.

Within this dual-process framework, two historically distinct approaches to the study of emotion can be distinguished. The first is the basic emotion approach. This approach describes the full spectrum of human emotions as a mixture of a limited set of basic emotions. It is focused on the output side of the emotion-generative process, namely the coordinated expression of complex patterns of behavior that comprise the observable, tangible, and socially impactful component of an emotional response. The second approach is the appraisal approach. Lazarus defines the appraisal approach as having two themes. The first is that emotion is a response to evaluative judgments or meaning; the second that these judgments are about ongoing relationships with the environment, namely how one is doing in the agenda of living and whether the encounter of the environment is one of harm or benefit (Lazarus, 1991). This approach has focused on the input side of the emotion-generative process, namely the processing of environmental stimuli that gives rise to the emotional response. These two approaches share two central assumptions. First, each of these approaches assumes that there are definable kinds of emotion (defined by the brain, or by the deep structure of situations). Second, these approaches assume that emotion generation is dominated by automatic processing (with regulation usually occurring after the fact).

Barret, Ochsner and Gross (2006) outlined the third approach as the modal model. Thiis modal model underlies lay intuitions about emotion (Barrett, Ochsner, & Gross, in press) and also represents major points of convergence among researchers and theoreticians concerned with emotion.

The basic emotion approach has helped to define emotion as a topic worthy of study in its own right, facilitating the development of empirical methods for examining facial (e.g., Ekman & Friesen, 1978), vocal (e.g., Scherer, 1986), autonomic (e.g., Cacioppo, Klein, Berntson, & Hatfield, 1993), and central (e.g., Davidson & Irwin, 1999) aspects of emotional responding. It has served as the de facto yardstick against which competing accounts of emotion are evaluated. The appraisal approach has helped to establish the importance of personal relevance and meaning in triggering emotional responses, and has attempted to unpack the notion of ballistic, automatic action programs into a more complicated set of both automatic and controlled processes that together contribute to the generation of an emotional response. Another important assumption of the modal model – namely that emotions are automatically generated -- has great intuitive appeal. Indeed, we 'see' evidence (or so we think) of highly automatic and stereotyped emotional responses in ourselves, in others, and in non-human animals (such as our dogs and cats). But are our emotions generated automatically as the modal model suggests, leading us this way or that depending upon which emotion has been elicited by a particular context? Barret, Ochsner and Gross (2006) think that in general, introspection does not give us privileged information regarding the causal mechanisms that give rise to our behavior (Nisbett & Wilson, 1977; Wilson & Dunn, 2004). Therefore, our experience of emotions as arising unbidden, and then taking us over, does not, in and of itself, constitute evidence that emotion generation is intrinsically automatic. To be fair, the original definition of automaticity was phenomenological in nature. Automatic processing was characterized by the absence of any subjective experience of control during thought, feeling, and behavior.

Finally another conceptualitation is through the Parallel distributed processing (PDP) models (also called neural networks or connectionist models). It is a neural network approach that stressed the parallel nature of neural processing, and the distributed nature of neural representations. It provided a general mathematical framework for researchers to operate in. The framework involved eight major aspects:

- A set of processing units, represented by a set of integers.
- An activation for each unit, represented by a vector of time-dependent functions.
- An output function for each unit, represented by a vector of functions on the activations.
- A pattern of connectivity among units, represented by a matrix of real numbers indicating connection strength.
- A propagation rule spreading the activations via the connections, represented by a function on the output of the units.
- An activation rule for combining inputs to a unit to determine its new activation, represented by a function on the current activation and propagation.
- A learning rule for modifying connections based on experience, represented by a change in the weights based on any number of variables.
- An environment which provides the system with experience, represented by sets of activation vectors for some subset of the units.

Scientists used to conceptualize the brain as a hierarchical set of specialized processing networks, but more recent neuroscience evidence suggests that the brain is a set of distributed, interacting networks. In a PDP model, networks of neuron-like units (called nodes) pass activation to one another in parallel. Nodes in a PDP model can represent information at any level of analysis. For example, in "localist" models, each node represents a type of psychological function or process (e.g., an instance of emotion). In "distributed" models, the psychological function or process is represented by a pattern of activation distributed across a group of nodes. The idea is that multiple brain circuits process different types of inputs in parallel, with the processing in each circuit limiting, shaping, and constraining the way in which the system achieves a single coherent "solution." For the purposes of this chapter, the "solution" is an instance of emotion that suits the particular goals of the individual and constraints of the context.

Early attempts to understand emotion using PDP ideas were inspired by appraisal models, and were therefore firmly grounded in the modal model. Appraisal models made explicit reference to ideas from parallel distributed processing (Scherer, 2001), and nonlinearity and neural network modeling (Frijda & Zeelenberg, 2001). For example, Wehrle & Scherer (2001) used a "black box" computational model that consisted of a set of formulas or algorithms to calculate emotional outputs (e.g., facial or vocal behaviors) on the basis of concrete input parameters (such as a profile of appraisals).

## CONCLUSION

In this chapter, we have reviewed the role of automatization on attitude; afterwards the role of automatization on social attribution and stereotyping and finally the role of automatization on emotions were presented.

Firstly we have seen that the classic studies highlight automatic forms of human responding. Like much of social psychology, these studies take the conscious control of behavior as a kind of backdrop, a taken-for-granted assumption that makes interesting news when it is shown to be in error. And in fact, this is a theme that has served social psychology well and no doubt will continue to do so as we march forward in our continued quest to test science against any and all sacred cows. As it turns out. however, this chapter has also revealed that the larger portion of mental processes, including those involved in social life, are characterized by control and automaticity.

We have also emphasized that control and automaticity both can be described broadly in terms of control theories. That is, both kinds of processes operate in the service of the individual's goals and purposes. Automatic processes furnish a massive amount of information to control judgment and decision processes more efficiently than would be possible with the slower and energy-demanding control processes alone.

The distinction between control and automatic mental processes is of critical importance in social psychology because it is the dividing line between what we purport to know about ourselves and what we do not. While the classic experiments in our field have shown us to be largely ignorant of the powerful effects that authority figures and majority opinion have on our behavior, at the same time they demonstrate our rather automatic ability to get along with others and function smoothly in a social organization, instead of as individuals acting in the service of our separate goals. Automatic processes constitute a broad undercurrent of life that keeps us connected to the world and behaving effectively on many planes in response to a welter of environmental and internal stimulation. Yet at the same time a thin thread of conscious control organizes these automatic processes and relates them to our goals and concerns.

In this chapter we have also seen the reflective-reflexive model based in neurocognitive systems and the techniques of neuroimaging that can make great contributions to the understanding of judgment and decision-making. The findings from this chapter as well as the other existing findings in social cognitive neuroscience are undoubtedly just the tip of the iceberg.

Finally we have seen the "modal model" of emotion that is important as an initial framework for the field. Using this framework, emotion researchers have developed methods that have yielded a large number of empirical findings. We have also seen early attempts to understand emotion using PDP ideas that were inspired by appraisal models, and were therefore firmly grounded in the modal model.

There are two important ideas in this background: that the field of emotion should be solely concerned with discrete kinds of emotion, and that the idea that emotions are typically generated automatically.

Concluding, there are a variety of internal representations that become activated automatically in the course of social life, such as attitudes, representations of social groups, anything to do with one's sense of self, and whatever is relevant to achieving one's current goals, Not only do these activated representations then play a major role in one's impressions and judgments about the situation, they also directly and nonconsciously affect one's behaviour in it.

## REFERENCES

[1]    Breckler, S. J., & Wiggins, E. C. (1992). On defining attitude and attitude theory: Once more with feeling. In A. R. Pratkanis, S. J. Breckler, & A. C. Greenwald (Eds.), *Attitude structure and function. Hillsdale* (pp. 407-427), NJ: Erlbaum.

[2]   Higgins, E. (1996). Knowledge activation: Accessibility, applicability, and salience. In E. T. iggins, & A. W. Kruganski (Eds.), Social Psychology, Handbook of basic principles (pp. 133-168). New York:Guilford Press.

[3]   Anderson, J. R. (1983). *The architecture of cognition.* Cambridge, MA: Harvard University Press.

[4]   Fazio, R. H. (1986). How do attitudes guide behavior? In R. M. Sorrentino & E. T. Higgins (Eds.), *The handbook of motivation and cognition: Foundations of social behavior* (pp. 204-243). New York: Guilford Press.

[5]   Eagly, A., & Chaiken, S. (1995). Attitude strength, attitude structure and resistance to change. In R. Petty & J. Kosnik (Eds.), *Attitude Strength* (pp. 413-432). Mahwah, NJ: Erlbaum.

[6]   Wegner, D. M., & Bargh, J. A. (1998). Control and automaticity in social life. In D. Gilbert, S. Fiske, & G. Lindzey (Eds.), *Handbook of social psychology* (pp. 446-496). Boston: McGraw- Hill.

[7]   Zajonc, R. B. (1968). Attitudinal effects of mere exposure. *Journal of Personality and Social Psychology, 9,* 1-28

[8]   Gordon, P. C., & Holyoak, K. J. (1983). Implicit learning and generalization of the "mere exposure" effect. *Journal of Personality and Social Psychology, 45,* 492-500.

[9]   Kunst-Wilson, W. R., & Zajonc, R. B. (1980). Affective discrimination of stimuli that cannot be recognized. *Science, 207,* 557-558.

[10]  Monahan, J. L., Murphy, S. T., & Zajonc, R. B. (2000). Subliminal mere exposure: Specific, general, and diffuse effects. *Psychological Science,11,* 462–466.

[11]  Perkins, A.W.,. Forehand M. R., and Greenwald A. G. (2006), Decomposing IAT-Measured Self-Associations: The Relative Influence of Semantic Meaning and Valence, *Social Cognition,* Forthcoming.

[12]  Cacioppo, J. T., Klein, D. J., Bernston, G. G., & Hatfiel, E. (1993). The psychophysiology of emotion. In: M. Lewis & J.M. Haviland-Jones (Eds), *Handbook of emotions,* (pp. 119-142). New York: Guilford Press.

[13]  Chaiken, S. (1980). Heuristic versus systematic information processing and the use of source versus message cues in persuasion. *Journal of Personality and Social Psychology, 39,*752-766.

[14]  Fazio, R. H. (1986). How do attitudes guide behavior? In R. M. Sorrentino & E. T. Higgins (Eds.), *The handbook of motivation and cognition: Foundations of social behavior* (pp. 204-243). New York: Guilford Press.

[15]  Fazio, R. H. (1990). Multiple processes by which attitudes guide behavior: the MODE model as an integrative framework. In M. Zanna (Ed.),

*Advances in experimental social psychology* (pp. 75–109). New York: Academic Press.

[16]  Petty, R. E., & Cacioppo, J. T. (1984). The effects of involvement on responses to argument quantity and quality: Central and peripheral routes to persuasion. *Journal of Personality and Social Psychology, 46,* 69-81.

[17]  Lieberman, M. D., (2003). Reflexive and Reflective Judgment Processes. A Social Cognitive Neuroscience Approach. In: J. P. Forgas, K. D. Williams, W. von Hippel, *Social Judgments: Implicit and Explicit Processes* (pp. 44-67). Cambridge University Press.

[18]  Ambady, N. & Rosenthal, R. (1993). Half a minute: Predicting teacher evaluations from thin slices of nonverbal behavior and physical attractiveness. *Journal of Personality and Social Psychology, 64,* 431-441.

[19]  Chen, M., & Bargh, J. A. (1999). Nonconscious approach and avoidance behavioral consequences of the automatic evaluation effect. *Personality and Social Psychology Bulletin, 25,* 215-224.

[20]  Word, C. O., Zanna, M. P., & Cooper, J. (1974). The nonverbal mediation of selffulfilling prophecies in interracial interaction. *Journal of Experimental Social Psychology, 10,* 109-120.

[21]  Nisbett, R. E. & Wilson, T. D. (1977). Telling more than we can know: Verbal reports non mental processes. *Psychological Review, 84,* 231-259.

[22]  Gilbert, D. T. (1989). Thinking lightly about others. Automatic components of the social inference process. In J. S. Uleman & J. A. Bargh (Eds.), *Unintended thought* (pp.189-211). New York: Guilford.

[23]  Heider, F., & Simmel, M. (1944). An experimental study of apparent behavior. *American Journal of Psychology, 57,* 243-259.

[24]  Winter, L., & Uleman, J. S. (1984). When are social judgments made? Evidence for the spontaneousness of trait inferences. *Journal of Personality and Social Psychology,47,* 237-252.

[25]  Langer, E. J., Blank, A. & Chanowitz, B. (1978). The mindlessness of ostensibly thoughtful action: The role of "placebic" information in interpersonal interaction. *Journal of Personality and Social Psychology, 36,* 635-642.

[26]  Lieberman, M. D., Gaunt, R., Gilbert, D. T., & Trope, Y. (2002). Reflection and reflexion: A social cognitive neuroscience approach to attributional inference. *Advances in Experimental Social Psychology, 34,* 199-249.

[27]  Carver, C. S, & Scheier, M. F. (1981). *Attention and self-regulation: A control theory approach to human behavior.* New York: Springer-Verlag.

[28]  Miller, G. A., Galanter, E., & Pribram, K. (1960). *Plans and the structure of behavior.* New York: Holt, Rinehart, & Winston.

[29]  Wiener, N. (1948). *Cybernetics: Control and communication in the animal and the machine*. Cambridge, MA: MIT Press.

[30]  Cherry, E.C. (1953). Some experiments on the recognition of speech with one and two ears. *Journal of the Acoustical Society' of America, 25*, 975-979.

[31]  Higgins, E. T., King, G. A., & Mavin, G. H. (1982). Individual construct accessibility and subjective impressions and recall. *Journal of Personality and Social Psychology, 43*, 35-47.

[32]  Wegner, D. M., & Vallacher, R. R.(1977). *Implicit psychology: An introduction to social cognition*. New York: Oxford University Press.

[33]  Fiske, S. T. (1980). Attention and weight in person perception: The impact of negative and extreme behavior. *Journal of Personality and Social Psychology, 38*, 889-906.

[34]  Hansen, C. H., & Hansen, R. D. (1988). Finding the face in the crowd: An anger superiority effect. *Journal of Personality and Social Psychology, 5*, 917-924.

[35]  Pratto, F., & John, O. P. (1991). Automatic vigilance: The attention-grabbing power of negative social information. *Journal of Personality and Social Psychology, 61*, 380-391.

[36]  Bargh, J. A. (1994). The four horsemen of automaticity: awareness, effciency, intention and control in social cognition. In R. Wyer Jr. & T. Srull (Eds.), *Handbook of social cognition* (2nd ed., pp. 1–40). Hillsdale, NJ: Erlbaum.

[37]  Brewer, M. B. (1988). A Dual Process Model of Impression Formation. In T.K. Srull and R.S. Wyer, Jr. (Eds.), *Advances in Social Cognition* (pp. 1-36). Hillsdale, N J: Erlbanm.

[38]  Fiske, S. T., & Neuberg, S. E. (1990). A continuum of impression formation, from category-based to individuating processes: Influences of information and motivation on attention and interpretation. In M. P. Zanna (Ed.), *Advances in experimental social psychology* (pp. 1-74). San Diego: Academic Press.

[39]  Macrae, C. N., Stangor, C., & Milne, A. B. (1994). Activating social stereotypes: A functional analysis. *Journal of Experimental Social Psychology, 30*, 370-389.

[40]  Fridja, N. H. (1986). *The emotions*. New York: Cambridge University Press.

[41]  LeDoux, J. E. (1996). *The emotional brain: The mysterious underpinnings of emotional life*. New York: Simon & Schuster.

[42]  Rolls, E. T. (1999). *The brain and emotion*. New York: Oxford University Press.

[43] Bruner, J. S. (1957). On perceptual readiness. *Psychological Review, 64,* 123-152.

[44] Haidt, J. (2001). The emotional dog and its rational tail: A social intuitionist approach to moral judgment. *Psychological Review, 108,* 814-834.

[45] Hogarth, R. H. (2001). *Educating intuition.* Chicago: University of Chicago Press.

[46] Lieberman, M. D. (2000a). Intuition: A social cognitive neuroscience approach. *Psychological Bulletin, 126,* 109-137.

[47] Bargh, J. A. (1999). The cognitive monster. In S. Chaiken & Y. Trope (Eds.), *Dual process theories in social psychology* (pp. 361-382). New York: Guilford Press

[48] James, W. (1890). *The principles of psychology.* New York: Henry Holt Co, Inc.

[49] Wilson, T. D., Dunn, D. S., Kraft, D., & Lisle, D. J. (1989). Introspection, attitude change, and attitude–behavior consistency: The disruptive effects of explaining why we feel the way we do. In L. Berkowitz (Ed.), *Advances in experimental social psychology* (pp. 123–205). San Diego, CA: Academic Press

[50] Wilson, F. A. W., Scalaidhe, S. P. O., & Goldman-Rakic, P. S. (1993). Dissociation of object and spatial processing domains in primate prefrontal cortex. *Science, 260,* 1955–1958.

[51] Macrae, C. N., Milne, A. B., & Bodenhausen, G. V. (1993). Stereotypes as energy-saving devices: A peek inside the cognitive toolbox. *Journal of Personality and Social Psychology, 66,* 37-47

[52] Dijksterhuis, A., & van Knippenberg A. (1996a). The knife that cuts both ways: Facilitated and inhibited access to traits as a result of stereotipe activation. *Journal of Experimental Social Psychology, 3,* 271-288.

[53] Pratto, F., & Bargh, J. A. (1991). Stereotyping based on apparently individuating information: Trait and global components of sex stereotypes under attention overload. *Journal of Experimental Social Psychology, 27,* 26-47.

[54] Bargh, J. A., Chen, M., & Burrows, L. (1996). Automaticity of social behavior: Direct effects of trait construct and stereotipe activation on action. *Journal of Personality and Social Psychology, 71,* 230-244.

[55] Anderson, J.R. (1983). *The architecture of cognition.* Cambridge, MA: Harvard University Press.

[56] Emde, R. N. ( 1984). Levels of meaning for infant emotions: A biosocial view. In K. R. Scherer & P. Ekman (Eds.), *Approaches to emotion* (pp. 77-107). Hillsdale, NJ: Erlbaum.

[57] Haviland, J. M., & Lelwica, M. (1987). The induced affect response: 10-week-old infants' response to three emotion expressions. *Developmental Psychology, 23*, 97-104.

[58] MacLean, P. D. (1993). Cerebral evolution of emotion. In M. Lewis & J. M. Haviland (Eds.), *Handbook of emotions* (pp.67-83). New York: Guilford.

[59] Ekman, P . (1992). An argument for basic emotions. *Cognition and Emotion, 6,* 169-200

[60] Barrett, L. F., Ochsner, K. N., & Gross, J. J. (2007). Automaticity and emotion. In J. Bargh (Ed.), *Automatic processes in social thinking and behavior.* New York: Psychology Press.

[61] Barrett, L. F., Tugade, M. M. & Engle, R. W. (2004). Individual differences in working memory capacity and dual-process theories of the mind. *Psychological Bulletin, 130,* 553-573.

[62] Chaiken, S. E. & Trope, Y. (1999). *Dual-process theories in social psychology.* New York: Guilford Press.

[63] Devine, P.G. (1989). Stereotypes and prejudice: Their automatic and controlled components. *Journal of Personality & Social Psychology, 56,* 5-18.

[64] Gilbert, D. T. (1991). How mental systems believe. *American Psychologist, 46,* 107-119.

[65] Gilbert, D. T. (1998). Ordinary personology. In: D.T. Gilbert & S.T. Fiske, (Eds.), *The handbook of social psychology,* (pp. 89-150). New York: McGraw-Hill.

[66] Power, M., Dagleish, T. (1997). *Cognition and emotion: From order to disorder.* Mahwah, NJ: Erlbaum.

[67] Schacter, D. L. (1997). The cognitive neuroscience of memory: perspectives from neuroimaging research. *Philos Trans R Soc Lond B Biol Sci, 352,* 1689-1695

[68] Sloman, S. A. (1996). The empirical case for two systems of reasoning. *Psychological Bulletin, 119,* 3-22.

[69] Smith, E. R. & DeCoster, J. (2000). Dual-process models in social and cognitive psychology: Conceptual integration and links to underlying memory systems. *Personality & Social Psychology Review, 4,* 108-131.

[70] Trope, Y. (1986). Identification and inferential processes in dispositional attribution. *Psychological Review, 93,* 239-257.

[71] Lazarus, R. S. (1991). *Emotion and adaptation.* Oxford: Oxford University Press.

[72] Ekman, P., & Friesen. W. V. (1978). *Facial action coding system: A technique for the measurement of facial movement.* Palo Alto, CA: Consulting Psychologists Press.

[73] Scherer, K. R. (1986). Vocal affect expression: A review and a model for future research. *Psychological Bulletin, 99,* 143-165.

[74] Davidson, R. J. & Irwin, W. (1999). The functional neuroanatomy of emotion and affective style. *Trends in Cognitive Sciences, 3,* 11-21.

[75] Wilson, T. D. & Dunn, E. W. (2004). Self-knowledge: Its limits, value and potential for improvement. *Annual Review of Psychology, 55,* 493-518.

[76] Scherer, K. R. (2001). Appraisal considered as a process of multilevel sequential checking. In: K.R. Scherer, A. Schorr, & T. Johnstone, (Eds.), *Appraisal processes in emotion: Theory, methods, research.* (pp. 92-120). London: London University Press.

[77] Frijda, N. H. & Zeelenberg, M. (2001). Appraisal: What is the dependent? In: K.R. Scherer, A. Schorr, & T. Johnstone, (Eds.), *Appraisal processes in emotion: Theory, methods, research.* (pp. 141-155). London: London University Press.

[78] Wehrle, T., Scherer, K. R. (2001).Toward computational modelling of appraisal theories. *Appraisal processes in emotion: Theory, methods, research.* 350–365.

*Chapter 7*

# THE ROLE OF AUTOMATIZATION
# IN CLINICAL SETTINGS

## ABSTRACT

Recent research has shown that automatic processes play an important role also in psychopathology and health related behavior. The purpose of this chapter is to present clinical application of the theoretical standpoint on automatization. Initially the deficit in automatization on intellectually disabled, dyslexic and ADHD subjects is presented; with reference to dyslexia, automaticity deficit has been attributed to left hemisphere neuro-cortical disruptions of the underlying neurological substrata that support developmental acquisition of reading subskills. Effects of inefficiently automatized phoneme-grapheme skills accumulate over time resulting in poor reading skills for the dyslexic patients, indeed the role of automatic deficit in ADHD is not well known. Secondly, the role of automatic processes in anxiety and in depression are presented. Depressed and anxious people generate negative products such as images, thoughts and inferences automatically. These automatic products, which are usually assessed via the verbalizations of the depressed person, would be the reflection of underlying automatic processes. Finally the role of automatic processes on addictive behavior is analyzed. The cognitive-behavioural model supposes that all of us have automatic intrusive thoughts, which are essential conditions for developing obsessions. These thoughts create attitudes – dysfunctional cognitive schemata. Anxiety during some stressful events can activate and strengthen these dysfunctional schemata. Patients try to get rid of anxiety by voluntary behavior (compulsions) such as addictive behaviours.

## AUTOMATIZATION DEFICIT IN DYSLEXIA

Dyslexia is a learning disability that manifests itself primarily as a difficulty with written language, and specifically with reading. It is separate and distinct from reading difficulties resulting from other causes, such as a non-neurological deficiency with vision or hearing, or from poor or inadequate reading instruction. Evidence suggests that dyslexia results from differences in how the brain processes written and spoken language. Although dyslexia is thought to be the result of a neurological difference, it is not an intellectual disability. Dyslexia is diagnosed in people of all levels of intelligence.

The role of automaticity in dyslexia is very important. In fact automaticity seems to be the core problem of dyslexia. Dyslexia research has implicated phonetic dysfunction in the phoneme-grapheme associations which underlie reading skills. Expert readers of normal developmental etiology have required less mental effort, faster processing speed, and reduced focal attention when applying reading subskills. Readers with dysphonia and poorly automatized reading subskills have required more time, mental effort, and attention.

Dyslexia automaticity deficit has been attributed to left hemisphere neuro-cortical disruptions of the underlying neurological substrata that support developmental acquisition of reading subskills. Effects of inefficiently automatized phoneme-grapheme skills accumulate over time resulting in poor reading skills that are detrimental to academic achievement. Kerry [1] (2007) conducted a research in which she uses neuropsychological methodology; in this research adults with dysphonetic dyslexia were selected for automaticity investigation via psychometrics and quantitative electroencephalography. Clinical group inclusion criteria included a current Learning Disability (LD) diagnosis in the reading skills domain and dysphonia evidence. LD and non-clinical (NC) adult volunteers were characterized by phonetic ability after administration of selected subtests of Woodcock Johnson, Revised, Achievement Tests, namely, Word Attack, Letter-Word Identification, and Passage Comprehension. Neuropsychological automaticity tasks included Rapid Automatized Naming, Rapid Alternating Stimuli, and Color-Word Stroop. Response time and Stroop-effect data were recorded. Passive electroencephalographic data collection technique allowed access to remnant cortical activity after the performance of automaticity tasks. Active task electroencephalographic data was collected during the performance of Congruent and Incongruent Stroop subtests. Automaticity in this LD sample was characterized by slower response times and comparable cortical activation to NC group; the LD group required more time, but used similar cortical activation to achieve the same outcome of the NC group. Response time data, related to speed of processing, demonstrated that the LD participants required more time to complete the neuropsychological tasks; however the differences of some response time results disappeared when covaried with age. Electrophysiological data, reflecting cortical activation and mental effort, demonstrated comparable between group activations during both the passive and active recording tasks for left frontal and temporal cortical target locations. Some support was found for the semantic processing interpretation for the Color-Word Stroop.

## AUTOMATIZATION DEFICIT IN ADHD

Another group that may cooccur with dyslexia and in which to investigate automatic deficit is the Attention-deficit/hyperactivity disorder (AD/HD or ADHD) group. ADHD is a neurobehavioral and a developmental disorder. It affects about 3 to 5% of children with symptoms starting before seven years of age. Global prevalence for children is approximately 5%, with wide variability dependent on research methodologies utilized in studies. It is characterized by a persistent pattern of impulsiveness and inattention, with or without a component of hyperactivity. ADHD is twice as common in boys as in girls. ADHD is generally a chronic disorder with 30 to 50% of individuals diagnosed in childhood continuing to have symptoms into adulthood. A review of the literature reveals a marked increase in the number of articles associated with comorbidity in child psychopathology in general and with ADHD in particular.

Between 50% and 80% of the children with ADHD meet also diagnostic criteria for other disorders [2]. Comorbidity between ADHD and developmental learning disorders is common. According to Barkley [3], 25% to 50% of children with ADHD have also LD.

The nature of the association between ADHD and LD, however, is uncertain. First, it must be cleared up if subjects with ADHD show the same characteristics as subjects with LD (DSM-IV, APA 1995) or if they manifest peculiar difficulties. Furthermore, the study has to discover if learning and attention problems are independent or if they are interrelated and usually coexistent [4]. There is, however, some evidence of the possibility that ADHD is a heterogeneous group of children that differ as regards to academic difficulties. Most of the children with ADHD do not show any strumental deficit but experience difficulty in problem solving, in writing and comprehension of and memory for interconnected complex information, such as the complicated events that a story usually tells.

The precise cause of attentional dysfunction in ADHD remains unclear. Some theorists focus on executive deficit [5, 6, 7, 8, 9, 10], others propose also a difficulty in automatizing the basic skills [12].

Executive dysfunction includes a deficit in the abilities implicated in goal-oriented processes, such as the initiation and the maintenance of efficient strategies and the programming and the planning of motor behaviour skills [11, 9]. They are involved in effortful mental processes.

Some researches on executive functions have been guided by the frontal metaphor, emphasizing the planning deficits that follow frontal injury [13, 14]. Other studies refer mainly to the disorder of working memory system [7] or to information processing [6].

Hypothesis that hyperactive children fail to develop automatic processing is less consolidate. Recent researches [12, 15, 16] suggest that ADHD children have no deficit in innate automatic tasks but they could exhibit trouble in acquired automatic skills [12].

With respect to comorbidity subjects, some theorists have investigated the neuropsychological functioning of ADHD for distinguishing subgroups with and without academic difficulties [17, 18, 12, 19].

Data suggest that children with ADHD/LD are characterized primarily by deficits in planning and problem-solving. Indeed, subjects with LD alone exhibit significantly poor performance on verbal and metaverbal measures, whereas subjects with ADHD alone are inferior in measures of executive functions [20].

Fabio and Viganò [21] conducted a study with the aim of testing the hypothesis that executive function deficits are partially due to a deficit in automatic processing at least. In order to answer this question, two experimental researches investigated automatic processes using two different paradigms. The first research studied automaticity in selective attention processes in normal and ADHD subjects, while the second analysed the cost and the benefits of selective automatization.

As seen above, in the second chapter, automatic processes can be observed in the difference of speed performance in basic skills in children with and without ADHD.

Subjects with ADHD could show greater cognitive effort in performing basic mental operations which require only limited allocations of attention capacity [22, 23].

The hypothesis that task inefficiency in ADHD children can be caused by EF deficit, as well as by automatic learning dysfunctions, has been investigated by

Merril's integrated procedure [24] and the procedure of perceptual and semantic identification [25, 26].

The first procedure [24] has investigated automatic and effortful processes by integration of a) the methodology of the functions of codification and b) the methodology of memory load. To inquire the functions of codification, classic methodology uses pairs of pictures.

The subjects are instructed to recognise, as quickly as possible, the two stimuli belonging to the same category. The methodology of memory load has been integrated with the methodology of the function of codification. Subjects must repeat a list of numbers during the codification task. Memory load has been manipulated by increasing or decreasing the memory set. The purpose was to measure the level of cognitive load which is sensitive to interference in ADHD and normal groups. Automatic processes, in fact, can be accomplished simultaneously with other cognitive processes without interference [25, 26, 27]. Thus, difference on interference of memory load could reflect a difference in automatic performance in subjects with and without ADHD.

Merril [24] has applied this integrated procedure with both subjects with mental retardation and normal ones. His data show that both the subjects with mental retardation and those normal are subjected to a cost in coding in the presence of a mnestic load. His research data are scarcely indicative with respect to the possible lack in automaticity relative to subjects with mental retardation, because also normal subjects show a cost in the process of coding in the presence of a memory load. To explain these data, Merril [24] speaks of coding processes *partially automated*, that is those processes which can be performed without attention resources; nevertheless, if some resources are supplied to them, these processes are performed better or more quickly.

Another result of Merril [24] is that the subjects with mental retardation show an increased cost when the coding is concerned with the research of a semantic identity in the stimulus with respect to the research of a physical identity. The author thinks that there may be two possible explanations of these data: the subjects with mental retardation either have fewer resources or they apply them in a less efficient way.

As far as the second procedure [25, 26] is concerned, one assumes that, when the selective attention is concentrated on the physical characteristics of the stimulus, the subject has to simply recognise the physical identity and use less knowledge resources. Under these circumstances, processes of coding of automatic type can rationalize the data.

When selective attention shifts on the semantic characteristics of the stimulus, the subject has to recognize the individual items, take them back to the categorial position and employ more knowledge resources. In this latter case, coding processes of controlled type can rationalize the data.

In the work by Fabio and Viganò [21] normal subjects with ADHD ("pure" or associated with an LD) have been examined, when performing selective attention in identifying visual stimulus [25]. The general aim was to understand whether the gaps discovered in the executive functions of the subjects with ADHD [5, 9, 11, 6, 7] are specific of executive functions or have to be ascribed, at least in part, to an unsuccessful access of the automatisms to the coding functions.

The logic underlying the work of Fabio and Viganò [21] was that the automatism of the coding process could be shown by the difference between the coding speed and the identification accuracy of the stimulus in the subjects with ADHD and with ADHD/LD and in the control [22, 23] of the two procedures: the physical and semantic identification procedure [25, 26] and the integrated procedure of Merrill [24] . The first aim of the study was to test the differences between physical and semantic level in children with ADHD, ADHD/LD and normal controls.

When selective attention is allocated on the physical characteristics of the stimulus, subjects use less knowledge resources, decrease the execution time and increase accuracy; when selective attention is allocated on the recognition of a stimulus at the semantic level, subjects employ more knowledge resources, increase execution time and decrease accuracy.

The second aim was to test the effortful/automatic hyphotesis for ADHD using the Merrill procedure [24]. The rationale was: if normal subjects and subjects with ADHD are able to perform the selection tasks equally well, both in the presence and in the absence of a memory load, then one can suppose that the selection is automatic; if, on the contrary, the subjects show a penalization due to the memory interference, then one can suppose that the selection is not automatic. In particular, if only the subjects of the group with ADHD show a low performance in the presence of a memory load, one can assume a specific deficit in ADHD in accessing the automatism. Participants in the study were selected from a database containing 520 children attending public primary schools in a district in Lombardy (Italy). The final sample included 10 children with ADHD (1 female, 9 males), 10 children with ADHD and LD (3 female, 7 males) and 10 normal controls (2 female, 8 males).

With respect to execution times, results show that the ADHD children were faster and the ADHD/LD children were slower than group controls in both experimental conditions. All groups increased their time of execution in a cognitive demanding task (semantic condition). Therefore, as the cognitive load increases, time of execution gradually increases in all groups.

Secondly, with respect to correct responses, all groups showed an inferior performance as regards semantic tasks, but the ADHD group's performance was worse than the other group's.

The factor *cognitive load* did not interact significantly with the execution of cognitive responses, in both experimental conditions.

Finally, regarding error rates, there was an increase in error rates across experimental conditions for all groups. The ADHD children had a greater increase in errors than the other groups.

Task performance was not sensitive to the level of cognitive load. No load significant effects were observed in task performance, in both experimental conditions.

ADHD subjects remained faster, in both experimental conditions, but they were also more variable and inaccurate in responding in semantic tasks.

In contrast to task efficiency (speed and accuracy), as found in the ADHD group in the physical condition, fast and inaccurate performance in task demanding cognitive resources can be explained in terms of impulsive responding: they keep "running" even if the task requires major allocation of attentional capacity.

These data are hard to be interpreted in the diatribe of automatic/controlled processes.

The main finding was that if effortful mental processes are requested, as in semantic tasks, requiring central information processing level, ADHD increase in error rate and decrease in correct responding. It can be said that ADHD subjects exhibit inefficiencies in effortful task because they show a deficit in executive functions, particularly, in self-monitoring processes but also that they display an inability in developing basic processing functions and they "lose" when a task becomes more difficult.

All subjects show a poorer performance when the cognitive load increases and, so, the data of this research do not allow us to assert that subjects with ADHD present a specific deficit of automatization.

In another work of Fabio and Viganò [21] another paradigm was used (see chapter 2), starting from the fact that automatization typically develops when the same stimulus has to be detected consistently over many trials.

The main aim of the research was to examine the automatic processes and the rigidity effect in a selective visual attention test: the Clock Test [30] .

Szymura, Slabosz and Orzechowski [31] used the Clock Test to study the speed-accuracy trade-off, automatization and rigidity relationships. Subjects had to detect the stimulus (an icon) representing hours on the clock (the dial). There were 40 signals and 40 distracting dials among stimuli. Other icons served as noise.

The icon of 4 o'clock was the target to detect. Subjects had 2 minutes to complete the test.

The index of automatization was calculated by the difference in correctness of selectivity mechanism between the third and the first trial and the difference in the number of errors between the third and the first trial. Automatization increased the correctness and reduced the errors.

In the study the same subjects of the first research were examined one month later.

The main aim was to evaluate if ADHD and LD/ADHD children have a lower index of automatization than normal children. The data analysis suggests that there were differences between the groups of the sample. The differences were due to selectivity automatization. In line with Shiffrin and Schneider [32] , the automatization effect was obtained by speed and accuracy performance measures.

With regard to the speed index, all the groups increased their speed in the response execution processes from trial 1 to trial 3. Furthermore, with reference to the accuracy index, the clinic groups showed a deterioration in the accuracy of their performance compared with controls.

In sum, findings indicate that both clinic groups present a lower automatization index than normal controls. Automatic processes require, in fact, an increase in response execution time and in accuracy.

Deficit or excess of automaticity may be a real problem in other pathologies too.


## AUTOMATIZATION DEFICIT IN INTELLECTUAL AND DEVELOPMENTAL DISABILITIES

Intellectual disability (ID) is characterized both by a significantly below-average score on a test of mental ability or intelligence and by limitations in the ability to function in areas of daily life, such as communication, self-care, and getting along in social situations and school activities. Children with intellectual disability can learn new skills, but they develop more slowly than children with average intelligence and adaptive skills.

Merrill [33]  reported that persons with intellectual disability (ID) are slower at learning a visual search task to automaticity relative to persons of the same age without ID. For persons without ID, automaticity develops most rapidly under conditions in which a response is always the same for a particular stimulus. The study of Merrill [33] was designed to investigate whether persons with and without ID are differentially sensitive to the influence of consistently mapped versus inconsistently mapped stimulus responses. The primary manipulation was the consistency between a particular stimulus and the response to that stimulus in a visual search task. Participants (with and without ID) searched displays of two, three, or four pictured objects to determine if a target was present. For half of the participants, the targets were always targets. For the other half, the targets became nontargets on 25% of the trials. Analyses focused on changes in response times associated with set size. Because automaticity allows for parallel processing, the elimination of significant effects of set size was taken as an index of the development of automaticity. Results indicated that inconsistent mapping significantly slowed the development of automaticity for the participants without ID but not for the participants with ID. Merrill conclude that these results can be discussed in terms of the role of inhibition processes in the development of automatic search and detection. The effectiveness of inhibition processes was compromised by the consistency manipulation. The effect of the consistency manipulation was greater for the participants without ID because they were presumed to be using inhibition processes more effectively during practice than did the participants with ID.

Also Dulaney and Ellis [22] in two studies examined the relationship between cognitive rigidity and cognitive inertia, with a total of 52 children and adults with mental retardation and 50 nonretarded individuals. Findings provide some support for the theory that there are age-related inherent structural differences leading to greater rigidity in older adults.

In another study Fabio and Cossutta [26] examined the possibility that sustained and selective attention differences between individuals with and without intellectual disability can be due to automatization deficit. Differences in stimulus encoding speed may reflect differences in the degree to which fundamental encoding processes operate automatically for individuals with and without mental retardation. For this reason a concurrent memory load procedure was used [34] combined with the selective attention methodology [24] to verify the theory of automaticity. The rationale was that if subjects perform equally well selective attention tasks with full memory load than they have really automatized basic processes. Subjects were 30 normal and 30 intellectually disabled who were selected on the basis of ratings from among 100 normal and 100 ID, the top 15 and the bottom 15 subjects in the ratings were designate as the good and the poor attenders. Subjects were presented with physical identity and name identity encoding while subjects retained a full memory load, half memory load and no memory load. Results indicated that subjects with mental retardation performed as well as normal subjects in no memory load condition, while they showed significant differences in full memory load condition. Moreover subjects intellectually disabled had a discontinuous encoding modality in sustained attention.

So, also in this case automaticity deficit seems to be confirmed.

## Automatic Processes in Anxiety

Anxiety is a psychological and physiological state characterized by cognitive, somatic, emotional, and behavioral components. These components combine to create an unpleasant feeling that is typically associated with uneasiness, fear, or worry.

Anxiety is a generalized mood state that occurs without an identifiable triggering stimulus. As such, it is distinguished from fear, which occurs in the presence of an external threat. Fear is related to the specific behaviors of escape and avoidance, whereas anxiety is the result of threats that are perceived to be uncontrollable or unavoidable. Anxiety is also a normal reaction to stress. It may help a person to deal with a difficult situation, for example at work or at school, by prompting one to cope with it. When anxiety becomes excessive, it may fall under the classification of an anxiety disorder.

Beck and Clarck [35] are interested in discovering the different perspective on anxiety and mainly the role of automatic thinking in anxiety.

McNally [36] recently offered a most thoughtful review on the role of automatic processes in anxiety. The distinction between automatic and controlled or strategic levels of control has played an important role in theories of attention, memory, and skill acquisition or performance [27, 28, 32, 37].

Wells and Matthews [38] considered "independence from attentional resources" and "insensitivity to voluntary control" the key criteria for automaticity. McNally [36] concluded that the processing bias in anxiety is automatic in terms of being involuntary and possibly unconscious but it is not resource or capacity-free. Controlled or strategic processes are considered qualitatively different from automatic processing. One of the hallmarks of strategic processing is its meaning assignment capabilities--its ability to provide meaningful interpretation of novel, complex information. Because of this, McNally [36] points out in his review that the propensity to inappropriately interpret innocuous stimuli or situations as threatening, a core cognitive process in anxiety disorders, probably depends on strategic, elaborative processing.

McNally [36] concluded that the view of automatic and, for that matter, strategic processing as unitary concepts has not been proven valid in social cognition studies that involve the processing of personally relevant and emotional information. That is, the various defining characteristics of automatic and strategic processing have not been found to reliably covary in these studies. Consequently some have argued that there are varieties of automaticity, others where all cognitive tasks involve varying amounts of automatic and strategic processing, and still others where automatic and strategic processing occur on a continuum [36].

Two further aspects of the automatic/strategic distinction are worth noting. First, the range of tasks and processes that have been characterized as automatic vary considerably, from experiments involving the subliminal presentation of discrete bits of information to the execution of highly complex tasks like driving a car, reading, make a decision or playing a musical instrument. Second, there is a dynamic nature to cognitive processing that involves movement back and forth between automatic and strategic processing. Many tasks acquire automaticity through practice, whereas other automatic, stereotypic tasks may succumb to controlled effortful intervention [39]. Given these considerations, the usefulness of the automatic/strategic processing distinction for understanding information processing in complex emotional states like anxiety can be questioned. McNally [36] noted that the development of pure-process experimental tasks may be very difficult if not impossible because most tasks involve a mixture of strategic and automatic processing. In sum, it may be more beneficial to consider the specific processing characteristics involved at the various stages of information processing in anxiety rather than to adhere rigidly to the automatic/strategic distinction.

In reply to McNally [36], Beck and Clarck [35] discuss a refined schema-based information processing model of anxiety that was originally presented in Beck et al. [40] . The authors are interested in the various characteristics that have distinguished automatic and strategic processing and in explaining how these processing characteristics define the cognitive basis of anxiety.

The cognitive model of anxiety first proposed by Beck et al. [40] is a schema-based information processing perspective that considers the erroneous or biased interpretation of stimuli as dangerous or threatening to an individual's physical or psychological well-being. Along with the selective processing of threat or danger stimuli, the anxious individual underestimates personal coping resources and the safety or rescue features in the environment. Furthermore, the distinction between normal and pathological anxiety is one of degree rather than kind because of the vital role that fear plays in the survival of the organism. The difference is that in pathological anxiety there is a biased or overestimated perception of danger which does not correspond to the exigencies of the internal or external environment, whereas in nonclinical anxiety states the estimation of threat corresponds more closely to the objective dangers in the environment. For example acute anxiety in response to repeated chest discomfort would be pathological for the young person with no previous history of coronary artery disease but it might be quite realistic for a middle aged man who recently suffered a myocardial infarct.

The cognitive model recognizes that anxiety consists of a complicated pattern of cognitive, affective, physiological and behavioral changes [35, 41].

As the authors underline, at the physiological level one finds autonomic hyperarousal in preparation for flight, fight, freezing or fainting. At the behavioral level there is (a) mobilization in order to escape or defend one's self against the perceived danger; (b) inhibition of risk taking behavior in an attempt to maximize safety; and (c) deactivation of motor responses resulting in avoidance and feelings of helplessness. At the subjective or affective level the individual feels frightened or apprehensive.

And finally, at the cognitive level anxiety involves: (a) certain sensory-perceptual symptoms such as feelings of unreality, hypervigilance and self-consciousness; (b) thinking difficulties such as poor concentration, inability to control thinking, blocking, and difficulty reasoning; and (c) conceptual symptoms like cognitive distortions, fear-related beliefs, frightening images and frequent automatic thoughts [40].

This complex cognitive-affective-physiological- behavioral pattern that we call anxiety arises from a particular three-stage information processing sequence that constitutes the very heart of the cognitive model of anxiety. Furthermore, it is the propensity of this information processing apparatus to inappropriately generate threat meaning assignments to innocuous stimuli that is the main problem that must be rectified in the treatment of anxiety disorders.

## Automatic Processes in Depression

*Depression* is a strong mood involving sadness, discouragement, despair, o hopelessness that lasts for weeks, months, or even longer.

In his cognitive model of depression, Beck [42] suggested that depressed people generate negative products such as images, thoughts and inferences automatically. These automatic products, which are usually assessed via the verbalizations of the depressed person, would be the reflection of underlying automatic processes. As Vázquez & Hernangómez [43] underline, different lines of empirical research have consistently found that, in fact, depressed persons have difficulties to plan, initialize and monitor complex goal-directed behaviors in the face of distracting negative information [44] . Thus, in a broader sense, depressed individuals seem to show a reduced executive control, which leads them, for example, to being unable to control or adequately redirect their attention when negative thoughts or images appear or even to retrieve rather over-general negative autobiographical memories.

In depressed persons as well as in depression-prone individuals, negative cognitions are more easily activated than in normal participants [45]. This distinction of a dual processing mechanism has proved to be a valuable tool to understand diverse findings in the literature on various cognitive processes in depression (attention, memory, thinking, etc.).

According to the differentiation of automaticity and control, the statement that biases in depression and anxiety operate on different processing levels that correspond to different cognitive tasks has become a dominant theme. Thus, it has often been stated that anxiety states are more closely related to biases in the automatic processing of threatening material (particularly reflected in attentional tasks) whereas depressive states are characterized by biases in operations of controlled processing (especially reflected in biases of memory)—e.g., Matt, Vázquez and Campbell [46] (1992). Depressed patients as well as recovered depressed patients seem to have difficulties to move attention away from negative information once it is presented [47]. Moreover, the data about this depression-versus-anxiety dichotomy reflecting different ways of processing are not as conclusive as has often been stated.

Several reports have demonstrated that depressed patients present impairments in situations that require conscious recollection of a studied episode (explicit memory tasks such as recall or recognition tasks) [48, 49, 50, 51]. On the other hand, most studies have revealed that performance on implicit memory tasks is unimpaired in individuals suffering from depression [50, 52, 53]. One interpretation of this dissociation between explicit memory deficits and preserved implicit memory performance is that depressed patients are impaired in their ability to use effortful (controlled) encoding and retrieval strategies, while their use of automatic processes is unimpaired [44] . However, this interpretation does not really take into account the fact that performance on any memory task (explicit or implicit) appears to result from the influence of both controlled and automatic processes. According to Jacoby, Toth, and Yonelinas [55] , performance on an explicit or an implicit memory task is not solely subtended by one kind of process: performance on any task is the result of the contribution of both controlled and automatic processes.

## Automatic Processes in Addictive Behaviour

Addictive behaviour is any activity, substance, object, or behaviour that has become the major focus of a person's life to the exclusion of other activities, or that has begun to harm the individual or others physically, mentally, or socially.

A person can become addicted, dependent, or compulsively obsessed with anything. Some researchers imply that there are similarities between physical addiction to various chemicals, such as alcohol and heroin, and psychological dependence to activities such as compulsive gambling, sex, work, running, shopping, or eating disorders.

Compulsive behaviours are rooted in a need to reduce tension caused by inner feelings a person wants to avoid or control. Compulsive behaviours are repetitive and seemingly purposeful and are often performed in a ritualistic manner.

The learning theory points out that obsessions are conditioned reflexes. The cognitive-behavioural model supposes that all of us have automatic intrusive thoughts, which are essential conditions for developing obsessions, but most of them are not stored. If they are connected with others – voluntary thoughts or behaviour, they can become aware and fixed. In the predisposed, the automatic thoughts can induce unusually strong or remaining tension, which activates the dysfunctional attitudes. These attitudes – dysfunctional cognitive schemata – are formulated during childhood, mainly by the influence of upbringing and social rules. Anxiety during some stressful events can activate and strengthen these dysfunctional schemata. Patients try to get rid of anxiety by voluntary behavior (compulsions).

Moreover there is evidence that the controlled regulatory processes are strongly weakened by the acute effects of alcohol, whereas more automatic, approach-oriented processes are not and can even be primed by drinking alcohol. Self regulation does not only depend on ability to inhibit appetitive tendencies; an individual should also be motivated to do so. Usually, the motivation to regulate addictive behaviours is low in adolescents, because adolescents often do not recognize their alcohol and drug use as problematic. The model presented by Wiers et al. [56] is primarily based on behavioral and electrophysiological research in human adolescents and young adults, with a focus on recent studies that have tried to assess relatively automatic cognitive motivational processes.

A paradigm used to highlight addictive behaviours related to automaticity is the Stroop test. As in the classical Stroop test [57], the task of the participant in the drug-Stroop test is to name the color of words presented on a computer screen (or classically on a card) while attempting to refrain from reading the color words themselves. Substance abusers do this more slowly for words that are related to their substance of abuse (e.g. "beer" is color named more slowly than "barn", among alcohol abusers). This "drug-Stroop" effect has now been demonstrated for many drugs of abuse [59, 59]. Basic research on attentional mechanisms distinguishes between different components of attention, including initial orienting to a stimulus and a later disengagement process [60]. The drug-Stroop test appears to primarily tap into the slower and more controlled disengagement process which is thought to be related to subjective craving [61, 58, 59] . Other tests of attentional bias may better tap into the early orienting aspect of attention, such as the visual probe task [60] . In this test, two pictures are shown simultaneously on a computer screen, one drug-related and the other not. After a brief interval these pictures disappear and a target stimulus that the subject must identify appears behind either the drug-related picture or the neutral picture. Drug abusers have often (but not always) been found to detect the target stimulus more quickly when it appears behind the drug-related picture compared to the neutral picture [62, 63].

As Wiers et al.[56] point out this finding suggests that drug-related cues capture early selective attention in drug abusers, which facilitates responding to a target appearing in the same location. Other promising tests of attentional bias also have been developed, such as the flicker paradigm for inducing change blindness [64, 65, 66]. During this task, a display with different objects (alcohol-related and neutral) is presented for 250 ms on a computer screen. Then a mask is briefly presented, after which the initial visual scene is presented again for 250 ms with one object changed. This object can be alcohol- (or drug-) related or not. This sequence is repeated until the participant detects the changing object. Jones et al. [65, 66] found that heavy drinkers detected an alcohol related change faster than a neutral change, a difference that was not seen in light drinkers. Jones et al. interpreted this result as evidence that heavy drinkers' attention is automatically grabbed and captured by alcohol-related cues, making it easier for them to detect changes associated with such cues and harder to detect changes in the neutral stimuli. Comparable results have been found for problem drinkers vs. social drinkers [64]. Wiers et al [56] think that this is an important issue for further research, as is the question of to what extent attentional bias is a causal factor in (or a close correlate of) the development of addictive behaviors [65, 66, 67, 68].

# CONCLUSION

In this chapter, we have reviewed the role of automatization on clinical settings. Problems of clinical interest can be due both to a deficit or excess of automatic processes. With reference to dyslexic and ADHD subjects problems arise from deficit in automaticity.

Dyslexia deficit has been attributed to effects of inefficiently automatized phoneme-grapheme skills accumulated over time resulting in poor reading skills that are detrimental to academic achievement. With reference to ADHD subjects, the main finding is that when effortful mental processes are requested, as in semantic tasks, requiring central information processing level, ADHD increase in error rate and decrease in correct responding. It can be said that they exhibit inefficiencies in effortful task because they show a deficit in executive functions, particularly, in self-monitoring processes, but also that they display an inability in developing basic processing functions and they "lose" when a task becomes more difficult. All subjects show a poorer performance when the cognitive load increases and, so, the data of this research do not allow us to assert that subjects with ADHD present a specific deficit of automatization.

With reference to the depressed and anxious subjects problems arise from excess of automaticity. Beck [42] suggested that depressed people generate negative products such as images, thoughts and inferences automatically. These automatic products, which are usually assessed via the verbalizations of the depressed person, would be the reflection of underlying automatic thinking. The distinction between controlled and automatic processes is probably a way to fruitful analysis also for anxious subjects. The results of some recent high-risk prospective studies show that the onset of anxiety and depression is more likely when there is a confluence of negative cognitive schemas (about oneself, the world, and the future) together with a tendency to process information ruminatively [69].

As Vázquez & Hernangómez [43] underline, different lines of empirical research have consistently found that depressed persons have difficulties to plan, initialize and monitor complex goal-directed behaviors in the face of distracting negative information [44]. Thus, in a broader sense, depressed individuals seem to show other than an excess of automaticity, a reduced executive control, which leads them, for example, to being unable to control or adequately redirect their attention when negative thoughts or images appear or even to retrieve rather over-general negative autobiographical memories.

Finally the role of automatic processes on addictive behavior has been analysed. Jones et al. [64] think that heavy drinkers' attention is automatically grabbed and captured by alcohol-related cues, making it easier for them to detect changes associated with such cues and harder to detect changes in the neutral stimuli.

## REFERENCES

[1]   Kerry, T., (2007). An investigation of automaticity in learning disabled (LD) and non-clinical adults. *Dissertation Abstracts International: Section B: The Sciences and Engineering, 68*, 1322.Riccio, C. A., Gonzalez, J. J. & Hynd G. W. (1994). Attention-Deficit Hyperactivity Disorder (ADHD) and Learning Disabilities. *Learning Disability Quarterly, 4*, 311-322.

[3]   Barkley, R. (1994). *ADD in the Classroom.* New York: Guilford Press.

[4]   Vio, C., Marzocchi, G. M. & Offredi, F. (1999). *Il bambino con deficit di attenzione/iperattività.* Trento: Erickson.

[5]   Shallice, T., Marzocchi, G. M., Coser, S., Del Savio, M., Meuter, R.F. & Rumiati, R.I. 2002). Executive function profile of children with Attention Deficit Hyperactivity Disorder (ADHD). *Developmental Neuropsychology, 21*, 43-71.

[6]   Sergeant, J. (1999). La valutazione del disturbo da deficit di attenzione/iperattività: il modello energetico-cognitivo. *A. I. D. A., 1.* Disponibile [online]: www. aidai.org

[7]   Barkley, R.A. (1997). Behavioral inhibition, sustained attention, and executive functions: constructing a unifying theory of ADHD. *Psychol Bull, 121*, 65–94.

[8]   Barkley, R. A. (1998). *Attention deficit hyperactivity disorder: A handbook for diagnosis and treatment* (2nd ed.). New York: Guilford.

[9]   Sechi, E., Corcelli, A. & Vasquez, P. (1998). Difficoltà esecutive e problemi di programmazione prassica nei bambini con Disturbi da Deficit dell'Attenzione con Iperattività. *Psichiatria dell'Infanzia e dell' Adolescenza, 65*, 187-195.

[10]  Swanson, J., Posner, M. I., Cantwell, D., Wigal, S., Crinella, F., Filipek, P. A., Emerson, J., Tucker, D. & Nalcioglu O. (1998). Disorder: symptom domain, cognitive processes and neural networks. In: R. Parasuram (Eds), *The Attentive Brain.* The MIT press.

[11] Pennington, B. F. & Ozonoff, S. (1996). Executive functions and developmental psychopathology. *Child Psychology and Psychiatry, 37,* 51-87.

[12] Ackerman, P. T., Anhalt, J. M., Holcomb, P. J. & Dykman, R. A. (1986). Presumably innate and acquired automatic processes reading problems. *Journal of Child Psychology and Psychiatry, 27,* 513-529.

[13] Grodzinski, G. M., & Diamond, R. (1992). Frontal lobe functioning in boys with attention deficit hyperactivity disorder. *Developmental Neuropsychology, 8,* 427-445.

[14] Levin, H. S., Eisenberg, H. M. & Benton, A. L. (1991). *Frontal lobe function and disfunction.* New York: Oxford University Press.

[15] Borcherding, B., Thompson, K., Kruesi, M., Bartko, J. J., Rapoport, J. & Weingartner H. (1988). Automatic and effortful processing in Attention Deficit/Hyperactivity Disorder. *Journal of Abnormal Child Psychology, 16,* 333-345.

[16] Ott, D. A. & Lyman, R. D. (1993). Automatic and effortful memory in children exibiting attention-deficit hyperactivity disorder. *Journal of Clinical Child Psychology, 22,* 420-427.

[17] Levi, G., Sechi, E. & Graziani, A. (1991). Disturbi dell'attenzione nei bambini con disabilità di apprendimento. *Psichiatria dell'Infanzia e dell'Adolescenza, 58,* 619-627.

[18] Denkla, M. (1996). A theory and model of executive function: A neuropsychological perspective. In G.R. Lyon & N.A Krasnegor (Eds) *Attention, memory and executive function* (pp.263-278). Baltimore: Paul H.Brookes

[19] Hazell, P. L., Carr, V. J., Lewin, T. J., Dewis, S. A. M., Heathcote, D. M. & Brucki, B. M. (1999). Effortul and automatic information processing in boys with ADHD and specific learning disorders. *Journal child psycology and psychiatry, 2,* 275 – 286.

[20] Penge, R. (2001). La comorbidità tra ADHD e DSA [online] http://sopsi.archicoop.it/ congres/cong_2001/simposi/abstract/36ab_3.htmFabio, R.A., & Viganò, A. (in press). Developmental and Cognitive Processing Deficits in ADHD: A Study of the Contribution of Automatic and Controlled Processes, *Journal of Learning Disabilities.*

[22] Dulaney, C. L. & Ellis, N. R. (1994). Automatized responding and cognitive inertia in individuals with mental retardation. *American Journal on Mental Retardation, 99,* 8-18.

[23] Logan, G. D., Taylor, S. E. & Etherton, J. L. (1996). Attention in the acquisition and expression of automaticity. *Journal of Experimental Psychology Learning, Memory, and Cognition, 3*, 620-638.

[24] Merril, E. D. (1992). Attentional resource demands of stimulus encoding for persons with and without mental retardation. *American Journal on Mental Retardation, 97, 1*, 87-98.

[25] Melnik, L. & Das, J. P. (1992). Measurement of attention deficit: correspondence between rating scale and tests of sustained and selective attention. *American Journal on Mental Retardation, 96, 6*, 599-606.

[26] Fabio, R. A. & Cossutta, R. (2001). Selezione automatica e modello multimodale in soggetti normali e con ritardo mentale. *Giornale italiano di psicologia, XXVIII 3*, 557–573.

[27] Hasher, L., & Zacks, R. T. (1979). Automatic and effortful processes in memory. *Journal of Experimental Psychology: General, 108*, 356-388.

[28] Posner, M. I., & Snyder, C. R. R. (1975). Attention and cognitive control. In R. L. Solso (Ed.), *Information processing and cognition: The Loyola Symposium* (55-85). Hillsdale, N J: Lawrence Erlbaum Associates.

[29] Lavie, N. (1995). Perceptual load as a necessary condition for selective attention. *Journal of Experimental Psychology Human Perception and Performance, 21, 3*, 451-468.

[30] Moron, M. (1997). Unpublished MA Thesis. Krakow: Jagiellonian University.

[31] Szymura, B., Slabosza, A. & Orzechowski, J. (2001). Some benefits and costs of the selectivity automatisation. *Atti XII conferenza annuale ESCOP*, Edimburgo.

[32] Shifrrin, R. M., & Schneider, W. (1977). Controlled and automatic human information processing: II. Perceptual learning, automatic attending, and a general theory. *Psychological Review, 84*, 127-190.

[33] Merrill, E.C. (2004). Consistent Mapping and Automatic Visual Search: Comparing Persons With and Without Intellectual Disability. Journal of Intellectual Disability Research, 48, 746-753.

[34] Logan, G. D. (1979). On the use of a concurrent memory load to measure attention and automaticity. *Journal of Experimental Psychology: Human Perception and Performance, 5*, 189-207.

[35] Beck, A. T., & Clark, D. A. (1997). An information processing model of anxiety: Automatic and strategic processes. *Behaviour Research and Therapy*, 35, 49-58.

[36] McNally, R. J. (1995). Automaticity and the anxiety disorders. *Behaviour Research and Therapy, 33*, 747-754.

138  Rosa Angela Fabio

[37] Schneider, W., & Shiffrin, R. M. (1977). Controlled and automatic human information processing:I. Detection, search, and attention. *Psychological Bulletin, 84*, 1-66.
[38] Wells, A., & Matthews, G. (1994). *Attention and emotion: A clinical perspective.* Hillsdale, NJ: Lawrence Erlbaum Associates.
[39] Sternberg, R. J. (1996). *Cognitive psychology.* Fort Worth: Harcourt Brace College Publishers.
[40] Beck, A. T., & Emery, G. (1985). *Anxiety disorders and phobias: A cognitive perspective.* New York: Basic Books.Clark, D. M., & Beck, A. T. (1988). Cognitive approaches. In C. Last & M. Hersen (Eds.), *Handbook of anxiety disorders* (pp. 362-385). Oxford: Pergamon Press.
[42] Beck, A.T. (1976). Cognitive therapy and the emotional disorders. New York: International University Press.
[43] Vázquez, C. & Hernangómez, L. (2008). Automatic and Controlled Processing in Depression. *International Encyclopedia of Depression*, 1-6.
[44] Hartlage, S., Alloy, L., Vázquez, C., & Dyckman, B. (1993). Automatic and effortful processing in depression. *Psychological Bulletin, 113*, 247-278.
[45] Lau, M. A., Segal, Z. V., & Wiliams, J. M. G. (2004). Teasdale's differential activation hypothesis: Implications for mechanisms of depressive relapse and suicidal behaviour. *Behaviour Research and Therapy, 42*, 1001-1017.
[46] Matt, J., Vázquez, C., & Campbell, K. (1992). Mood-congruent recall of affectively toned stimuli: A meta-analytic review. *Clinical Psychology Review, 2*, 227-256.
[47] Joormann, J., & Gotlib, I. H. (2007). Selective attention to emotional faces following recovery from depression. *Journal of Abnormal Psychology, 116*,1, 80-85.
[48] Jermann, F., Van der Linden, M., Adam, S., Ceschi, G., Perroud, A.(2005). Controlled and automatic uses of memory in depressed patients: effect of retention interval lengths. *Behaviour Research and Therapy, 43*, 681–690.
[49] Channon, S., Baker, J. E., & Robertson, M. M. (1993). Effects of structure and clustering on recall and recognition memory in clinical depression. *Journal of Abnormal Psychology, 102*, 323–326.
[50] Danion, J. M., Willard-Schroeder, D., Zimmermann, M. A., Grange, D., Schlienger, J. L., & Singer, L. (1991). Explicit memory and repetition priming in depression. Preliminary findings. *Archives of General Psychiatry, 48*, 707–711.

[51]  Hertel, P. T., & Rude, S. S. (1991). Depressive deficits in memory: focusing attention improves subsequent recall. *Journal of Experimental Psychology: General, 120,* 301–309.

[52]  Denny, E. B., & Hunt, R. R. (1992). Affective valence and memory in depression: dissociation of recall and fragment completion. *Journal of Abnormal Psychology, 101,* 575–580.

[53]  Hertel, P. T., & Hardin, T. S. (1990). Remembering with and without awareness in a depressed mood: evidence of deficits in initiative. *Journal of Experimental Psychology: General, 119,* 45–59.

[54]  Watkins, P. C., Mathews, A., Williamson, D. A., & Fuller, R. D. (1992). Mood-congruent memory in depression: emotional priming or elaboration? *Journal of Abnormal Psychology, 101,* 581–586.

[55]  Jacoby, L. L., Toth, J. P., & Yonelinas, A. P. (1993). Separating conscious and unconscious influences of memory: measuring recollection. *Journal of Experimental Psychology: General, 122,* 139–154.

[56]  Wiers, R. W., Bartholow, B. D., van den Wildenberg, E., Thush, C., Engels, R. C.M.E., Sher, K. J., Grenard, J., Ames, S. L. & Stacy, A. W. (2007). Automatic and controlled processes and the development of addictive behaviors in adolescents: A review and a model. *Pharmacology, Biochemistry and Behavior, 86,* 263–283.

[57]  Stroop, J. R. (1935). Studies of interference in serial verbal reactions. *J Exp Psychol, 18,* 643–62.

[58]  Cox, W. M, Fadardi, J. S. & Klinger, E. (2006a). Motivational processes underlying implicit cognition and addiction. In: R.W. Wiers & A.W, Stacy (Eds), *Handbook of implicit cognition and addiction* (253-266). Thousand Oaks CA: SAGE.

[59]  Cox, W. M, Fadardi, J.S. & Pothos, E. M. (2006b). The addiction–Stroop test: theoretical considerations and procedural recommendations. *Psychol Bull, 132,* 443–76.

[60]  [60]       Field, M., Mogg, K. & Bradley, B. P. (2006). Attention to drug-related cues in drug abuse and addiction: component processes. In: R.W. Wiers & A.W. Stacy (Eds), *Handbook of implicit cognition and addiction* (pp. 45-57). Thousand Oaks CA:SAGE.

[61]  Stormark, K.M., Laberg, J. C., Nordby, H. & Hugdahl, K. (2006). Alcoholics' selective attention to alcohol stimuli: automated processing? *J Stud Alcohol,61,*18–23.

[62]  Lubman, D. I., Peters, L. A., Mogg, K., Bradley, D. P. & Deakin, J. F. W. (2000). Attentional bias for drug cues in opiate dependence. *Psychol Med, 30,* 169–75.

[63] Townshend, J. M. & Duka, T. (2001). Attentional bias associated with alcohol cues: differences between heavy and occasional social drinkers. *Psychopharmacology,157,1,* 67–74.

[64] Jones, B. C., Jones, B. T., Blundell, L. & Bruce, G. (2002). Social users of alcohol and cannabis who detect substance-related changes in a change blindness paradigm report higher levels of use than those detecting substance-neutral changes. *Psychopharmacology,165,* 93–96.

[65] Jones, B. T., Jones, B. C., Smith, H. & Copley, N. (2003a). A flicker paradigm for inducing change blindness reveals alcohol and cannabis information processing biases in social users. *Addiction, 98,* 235–44.

[66] Jones, B. T., Jones, B. C., Smith, H. & Copley, N. (2003b). A flicker paradigm for inducing change blindness reveals alcohol and cannabis information processing biases in social users. *Addiction, 98,* 235–44.

[67] Jones, B. T., Bruce, G., Livingstone, S. & Reed, E. (2006). Alcohol-related attentional bias in problem drinkers with the flicker change blindness paradigm. *Psychol Addict Behav,20, 2,* 171–177.

[68] De Jong, P. J., Kindt, M. & Roefs, A. (2006). Changing implicit cognition: findings from experimental psychopathology. In: R. W. Wiers & A. W. Stacy (Eds), *Handbook of implicit cognition and addiction* (pp.425-437). Thousand Oaks CA: SAGE.

[69] Field, M. & Eastwood, B. (2005). Experimental manipulation of attentional bias increases the motivation to drink alcohol. *Psychopharmacology,183,* 350–357.

[70] Wiers, R. W., De Jong, P. J., Havermans, R. & Jelicic, M. (2004). How to change implicit drugrelated cognitions in prevention: a transdisciplinary integration of findings from experimental psychopathology, social cognition, memory and learning psychology. *Subst Use Misuse, 39,* 1625–1684.

[71] Wiers, R. W., Cox, W. M., Field, M., Fadardi, J. S., Palfai, T. P., Schoenmakers, T. & Stacy, A. W. (2006b). The search for new ways to change implicit alcohol-related cognitions in heavy drinkers. *Alcohol Clin Exp Res, 30,* 320–31.

[72] Alloy, L. B., Abramson, L. Y., Whitehouse, W. G., Hogan, M. E., Panzarella, C., & Rose, D. T. (2006). Prospective incidence of first onsets and recurrences of depression in individuals at high and low cognitive risk for depression. *Journal of Abnormal Psychology, 115,* 145-156.

# CONCLUSION

We have surveyed several particularly active research areas within the context of the attention and performance tradition, focusing on studies concerning automatic and controlled processes.

We revised the major empirical paradigms in which these phenomena are explored. In chapter three the growing body of functional anatomical studies, which examine the brain structures activated in the context of controlled and automatic behaviour has been presented.

At the end of the first part a question regarding the costs and benefits of controlled and automatic processes has been proposed. Beginning the second part of the book, chapter five was the core chapter of the book; it explored ways of accessing complex thinking through automatization. It is suggested that with training, people can operate without attentional control and improve their logical abilities. The theme of operational implications continued in the next chapter when we affirmed that controlled and automatic processing have very serious consequences for a person's phenomenal experience and for one's relations with others. Finally the book ended with the application of both concepts, automatic and controlled processes, on clinical populations.

As seen above, in chapter five we presented a model in which I considered that through automatization it is possible to have access to more complex cognitive processes. In this model in any starting step of a task, initially we use controlled processes of attention to codify and learn information; so performance is slow, awkward and prone to errors. We can say that the full amount of our memory load is engaged, we can also say, in other words, that all our cognitive resources are engaged to complete the new learning.

As training proceeds, performance requires less vigilance, becomes faster and errors decrease, a transformation that can be defined as "automatization". With learning, the attentional strategies that once needed control become automatic. We can have access to a more complex level. Again initially controlled processes are required, and as training proceeds, performance requires less vigilance, becomes faster and errors decrease; again we see automatization. In other words, with learning, the attentional strategies that once needed control become automatic. And so on. The infinity symbol, at the top of the figure related to the model, means that there is no limit to the possibility to accessing increasing stages of complex thinking.

To explain what happens in each level, before automatization arises, the catastrophe model is employed. It is assumed that learning occurs through accumulated exposure to stimulus. If one assumes that performance improves only gradually a first, the S-shaped learning curve is appropriate:

$$\text{Ln RT (t)} = (1/M) \{ A + B \text{ Ln (t)} + C \text{ Ln } (t^2) + D \ln (t^3) \}$$

where M, A, B, C, and D are empirically determined. In any case the learning process converges to a point where there is little or no schema development. Dynamically, as Flor and Dooley (1999) state, in the learning process is to a point attractor; in statistic convergence is indicated by weak stationarity: that means that mean, variance and covariance remain constant and independent of time. Convergence is in part indicated by the lack of divergence or chaotic dynamic, but initial stages of when the brain is testing competing schema both divergence and convergence would be present. The presence of divergent dynamic is an indication of chaos. The output of a chaotic system is point by point unpredictable, but forms a recognizable pattern over time if observed properly. The discovery of chaos leads to a rejection of the random hypothesis.

So, the early stages of the learning process is by a chaotic dynamic. This may be because the brain is searching for the optimal chunking pattern. This type of chaotic search has been found also in numerous studies of neuron level activity in which it is known that sensitivity to initial conditions allows amplification of small fluctuations, they may create and may destroy informations. As performance on the learned task converges, a state of mastery is achieved and so, further exposure to the learning task results in chunking rather than in improvement in performance. Less and less effort is required, and process and action become automatic. Thus chunking may explain why tasks can become automatic. Chunking may tend to follow a model of puntuacted equilibrium, where long periods of stasis are interrupted by short periods of rapid change. This is similar to the evolutionary dynamic seen in genetic systems and also observed in human societal development. It is similar also to the dynamic of the catastrophe model.

Several questions remain open. For some time it seemed perfectly reasonable to define an automatic process simply as having qualities opposite to those of conscious control, but this approach has proven problematic. Unlike the properties of conscious control, those of automatic processes do not hang together in an all-or-none fashion.

There are several features which must be jointly present in a psychogical process for it to count as an instance of conscious Control. The first open question is: how does the brain process sensory information consciously, and how does conscious attention stabilize memory? Second, what studies on the neural basis of automatic and controlled processes tell us? May be the studies on the neural basis, even though well conducted, show simply the co- appearance of both phenomena, not a causal relationship. Third, can the catastrophe model explain how unconscious and conscious mental processes relate to one another in people?

# INDEX

maladaptive, 76
males, 130
management, 27, 73, 76
manipulation, 14, 34, 85, 133, 146
mapping, 14, 35, 36, 44, 48, 61, 82, 133
mask, 38, 46, 49, 139
masking, 50
mastery, 96, 148
Matrices, 69
matrix, 116
meanings, 7, 8
measurement, 124
measures, 43, 52, 95, 109, 128, 132
medial prefrontal cortex, 57, 65
mediation, 120
membership, 74, 110
memory deficits, 137
memory performance, 137
memory retrieval, 18, 19, 46, 49, 89
men, 74
mental ability, 132
mental activity, 14
mental life, 1
mental processes, 29, 77, 117, 120, 128, 131,
   140, 149
mental representation, 24, 107
mental retardation, 41, 51, 129, 133, 142, 143
messages, 109
meta-analysis, 57, 65
metaphor, 128
missiles, 84
MIT, 29, 68, 78, 101, 103, 104, 121, 141
modalities, 70
modality, 134
modeling, 28, 104, 117
models, 21, 24, 26, 27, 67, 74, 86, 95, 104,
   108, 109, 114, 116, 117, 118, 123
modulation, 51
modules, 26, 27, 59
monkeys, 56, 60, 68
mood, 106, 134, 136, 145
moral judgment, 122
motion, 20, 112, 114
motivation, 30, 89, 101, 109, 119, 121, 138,
   146

motor skills, vii, 92
motor system, 111
movement, 124, 135
multivariate, 104

**N**

naming, 22, 32, 36, 90
National Academy of Sciences, 51
negative valence, 107
negativity, 61, 62, 63, 65, 70
network, 25, 27, 39, 61, 67, 95, 106, 116, 117
neural network, 57, 95, 116, 117, 141
neuroanatomy, 52, 124
neurobehavioral, 127
neuroimaging, 57, 58, 105, 118, 123
neurons, 57, 60, 68, 94
neuroscience, 44, 66, 101, 116, 118, 120, 122,
   123
New York, 29, 30, 66, 67, 68, 69, 101, 103,
   119, 120, 121, 122, 123, 141, 142, 144
nodes, 39, 95, 106, 116
noise, 42, 75, 110, 132
non-clinical, 126, 141
nonconscious, 29
non-human, 115
nonverbal, 109, 120
normal, 41, 52, 126, 128, 129, 130, 132, 133,
   134, 135, 137
normal children, 132
normal development, 52, 126
norms, 73
novel stimuli, 19, 66, 106
nuclei, 60, 66
nucleus, 57

**O**

observations, 74, 90
older adults, 133
one dimension, 20
organ, 1, 118
organism, 12, 135
orientation, 56
overload, 17, 113, 122

## T

**U**

**V**

**W**

**Y**